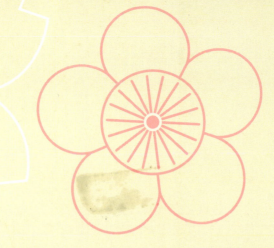

FACIAL FITNESS

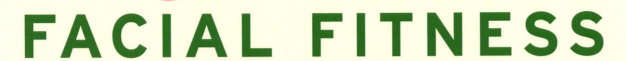

FACIAL FITNESS

DAILY EXERCISES & MASSAGE TECHNIQUES FOR A HEALTHIER, YOUNGER LOOKING YOU

PATRICIA GOROWAY
Foreword by Dr. Richard H. Keller, DDS, MPS

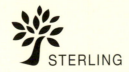

STERLING

New York / London
www.sterlingpublishing.com

STERLING and the distinctive Sterling logo are registered trademarks of Sterling Publishing Co., Inc.

The Library of Congress has cataloged the hardcover edition as follows:
Goroway, Patricia.
Facial fitness : daily exercise and massage techniques for a healthier, younger looking you / Patricia Goroway.
p. cm.
ISBN-13: 978-0-7607-8094-7 (alk. paper)
ISBN-10: 0-7607-8094-3 (alk. paper)
1. Facial exercises.   2. Face—Massage.   3. Beauty, Personal.   I. Title.

RA778b.G67 2006
646.7'2—dc22
2006015945

5   7   9   10   8   6   4

Published by Sterling Publishing Co., Inc.
387 Park Avenue South, New York, NY 10016
© 2010 by Patricia Goroway
Distributed in Canada by Sterling Publishing
c/o Canadian Manda Group, 165 Dufferin Street
Toronto, Ontario, Canada M6K 3H6
Distributed in the United Kingdom by GMC Distribution Services
Castle Place, 166 High Street, Lewes, East Sussex, England BN7 1XU
Distributed in Australia by Capricorn Link (Australia) Pty. Ltd.
P.O. Box 704, Windsor, NSW 2756, Australia

Printed in China
All rights reserved

ISBN: 978-1-4027-8046-2

For information about custom editions, special sales, premium and
corporate purchases, please contact Sterling Special Sales
Department at 800-805-5489 or specialsales@sterlingpublishing.com.

DEDICATION

This book is dedicated to my father, Ronald James Connolly, 1935–2006.

ACKNOWLEDGMENTS

I would like to thank the many friends, colleagues, editors, and medical professionals who have assisted me in writing this book, including:

Nathaniel Marunas, Betsy Beier, and Devorah Klein at Sterling Publishing for their skill and support, and for making this project a reality.

Dr. Richard Keller for introducing me to the possibilities of facial exercising.

My father, Ronald Connolly for his love, knowledge, and support, and for making me aware of the questionable ingredients used in skin care products.

Erik, Grace, and Joanna for their friendship, love, and encouragement through a difficult time.

David, for sharing his brilliant ideas and insights. And to my sons, Travis and Hunter, for their love, and for making me so proud.

All who contributed to this work with their personal and professional knowledge. Their input is greatly appreciated.

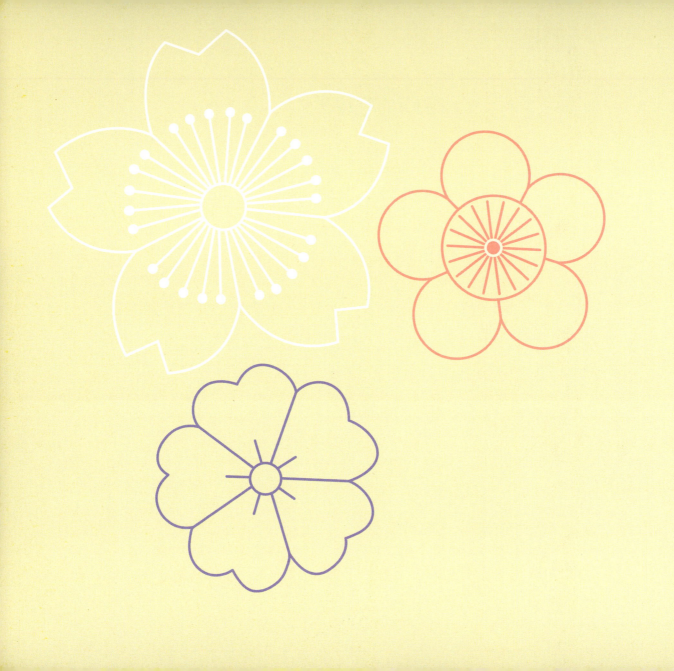

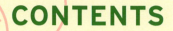

CONTENTS

FOREWORD

AS A BIOLOGICAL dentist who focuses on head and neck pain and temporomandibular joint (TMJ) dysfunction, nothing is more gratifying than patients who ultimately become pain-free, and who embrace healthy habits that ensure they remain pain-free. I have found that recommending exercises as prescribed in Patricia Goroway's *Facial Fitness* is necessary to support this healing process. Not only do Ms. Goroway's detailed exercises and regimens promote natural healing and muscle tonus, they result in healthier skin and a tighter face, giving readers a more youthful appearance.

Whether you have sought surgical or non-surgical solutions for maintaining the appearance of your early years, this book's holistic, noninvasive approach will help rejuvenate your face and neck. Readers will find that the detailed and clear instructions easily facilitate a continued commitment to vibrant, glowing, and—most importantly—well-toned skin. I know: I have been practicing the exercises and massage techniques since I received the manuscript!

In addition to exercises, massage techniques, and a regimen to support the muscles of the face and neck, *Facial Fitness* provides crucial information about utilizing well-chosen, natural skin products that will achieve the best results for your skin. (All beauty products are not alike!) It will also introduce you to high standards of integrating good lifestyle choices such as drinking plenty of clean, non-chemically tainted water; consuming vitamins, minerals, and healthful food; and aerobically exercising all your muscle groups; which will promote the body's own capabilities to heal, rejuvenate, and obtain optimal health.

Now that *Facial Fitness* is available, I intend to recommend it to my temporo-mandibular dysfunction patients, who I am sure will benefit immensely from the step-by-step explanations for the exercises and massages. During my last forty years of practicing dentistry, I have found that people with good physical and mental health radiate youthfulness and vitality. So whether you are using the exercises and massage techniques for rehabilitation, simple toning to decrease wrinkles, or to maintain surgical alterations, *Facial Fitness* is sure to be very useful to your physical and emotional health.

—*Dr. Richard H. Keller, DDS, MPS*

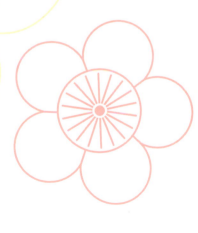

INTRODUCTION

Years ago, after what was to be a life-changing automobile accident, I discovered the amazing effects that exercising the muscles of the face and neck had on the injuries I sustained during that accident. The experience was life-changing because it left me with a newfound recognition that it is often possible to find alternatives to the generally prescribed course of treatment. I suffered a debilitating injury involving my neck and my temporomandibular joint, or TMJ. I had incredibly sharp pain that ran across my face. My bottom jaw was left misaligned and glided to one side when I opened my mouth. It popped and cracked so loudly whenever I tried to eat solid food that the sound was audible to others around me.

A surgical specialist advised me that surgery was the only way to minimize my pain and restore normal form and function to my face. The proposed procedure required incisions to be made on both sides of my face (possibly leaving scars) in an attempt to tighten the muscles and ligaments and hopefully relieve the pain and correct the misalignment. There was no guarantee this procedure would work, and my mouth would be wired shut, which meant that I would be on a strictly liquid diet for a sustained period of time.

Thankfully, I sought a second opinion and was directed to a physician specializing in facial and cranial rehabilitation. His approach included treating the injuries with a series of strengthening exercises to help eliminate the pain and correct the misalignment naturally. As clumsy and difficult as they were to perform, the exercises really worked. Within a month the pain was gone. But what happened next was truly amazing: not only were the muscles that had been directly affected by the injury toned, tightened, and pain free, but so were the surrounding muscles.

I have always been acutely aware of the importance of good skin-care. When I was a child, my father was in the cosmetics and skin-care industry and had access to the latest research and developments in the field. From an early age, he taught me the importance of good skin-care and how to be aware of the ingredients that cosmetic products contain.

As an adult, I became even more interested in the field and paid close attention to the latest information and so-called "breakthrough" skin-care and cosmetic products and procedures. When I visited my dermatologist for various conditions, I made a point of asking her opinion about the latest products and options. The options sounded promising, but somewhat limited. After all, just applying moisturizer to our bodies does not produce toned muscles. I was sure there was more that people could do to improve their skin by toning the muscles underneath.

After my accident, I began to conduct even more detailed research about the face, and in particular, its muscles, by consulting medical specialists, reading medical journals, and learning everything I could about how and why these muscles respond so well to exercise. I soon discovered that the muscles of the face and neck are all connected in a striated, quilt-like structure that lies just below the surface of the skin. Interwoven by fibers, the muscles are attached to each other, to the bone, and to the skin. They work synergistically to help you do everything from smiling and frowning to chewing, whistling, breathing, and even swallowing. Every expression you make, as well as every emotion and reaction you experience, is displayed on your face because of the connection of these muscles to specific cranial nerves whose nuclei lie within the brain stem.

The science is complicated, but here's the bottom line: scientists believe that the muscles of the face and neck are unique because of their involuntary link to your emotional processes. They also believe that no other animal has evolved as complex a set of facial muscles as humans have.

Scientists believe that the muscles of the face and neck are unique because of their involuntary link to your emotional processes.

I was fascinated by the information I discovered and the results I achieved by doing the facial exercises recommended to me by my doctor. I decided that I wanted to develop a series of exercises that would target all the muscles of the face and neck and create a complete facial exercise program. So, I continued my research. I studied anatomy and asked lots of questions to anyone I came across in the medical, health, or beauty industry. The common theme I came across again and again was that exercising the muscles of the face and neck is extremely beneficial to laying the groundwork for a youthful complexion.

So, how does it work? Through my research, I learned that the supply of blood to a contracting muscle is ten times greater than it is to a muscle at rest. This fresh blood supply delivers vital oxygen and nutrients to the skin and revitalizes the tissues. It is an all too common practice for people, especially women, to attempt to tighten the skin over a slack underlying structure through the use of plastic surgery, only to have the inevitable effects of gravity cause the face to appear droopy once again.

With that in mind, I began to adapt the basic maneuvers I had learned during my rehabilitation into a series of facial exercises that would work many of the fifty-seven muscles of the face and neck. The results were phenomenal. Not only were my muscles becoming toned and tightened, but fine lines and wrinkles began to fill in, erasing the signs of aging. And that was only the beginning. I then developed a series of facial massage techniques that were specifically designed to accompany and enhance the facial exercise program. After years of research and fine-tuning, the Facial Fitness program was born.

I have been teaching the Facial Fitness system since 1999 to individuals, organizations, readers, and health and skin-care professionals, and have also been busy certifying countless numbers of Facial Fitness instructors around the world.

These instructors are also certified to teach and share the secrets of Facial Fitness's Rehabilitation Program, which was designed to help correct facial imbalances and conditions of the face and neck such as TMJ and Bell's palsy. For more information on this unique certification, and the Facial Fitness system in general, please visit our website at www.facialfitnesssystems.com.

So what has made the Facial Fitness program so incredibly effective and successful for all these years? First and foremost, it is the fact that we address the complex combination of factors that affect the skin by utilizing a unique four-pronged approach to skin rejuvenation:

- Facial exercise, using movements to revitalize and strengthen your facial muscles.

- Facial massage, using rubbing and kneading to alleviate stress, increase circulation, and improve the skin's ability to eliminate toxins.

- Nutritious diet, using wholesome foods to see fast results for fabulous, healthy skin.

- Healthy skin-care, using nourishing methods to improve the tone and texture of skin while preventing further damage.

Many people resort to cosmetic procedures to improve their appearance. However, as I myself found out, these procedures are temporary and can be quite costly, especially when you have to keep repeating them every few months to maintain the desired effects. So, why not try exercising first? You will see the change in your appearance almost immediately, and in time you will be able to sculpt your face as you would your body, through strength training, to achieve a more youthful, radiant look.

I've never been afraid to try new things, but I have usually preferred a natural approach to improving my health and appearance whenever possible. I believe in seeking out alternative methods for improving one's health and appearance without the use of surgery. Developing the Facial Fitness program was simply a logical progression for me to rehabilitate, improve, and maintain a healthy, youthful complexion.

Because the muscles of the face and neck are smaller than most other muscles in the body, they respond very quickly to exercise. As a result, my facial exercise regimen,

in conjunction with the facial massage techniques I've incorporated into the program, will erase years of aging in just weeks. And, with regular practice, you will maintain that youthful, healthy look for years to come.

. . . you will be able to sculpt your face as you would your body, through strength training, to achieve a more youthful, radiant look.

My goal is to offer an alternative to costly and potentially risky procedures (after all, every surgery carries risks, no matter how well established the procedure is) and to help you cultivate a more natural-looking beauty by simply exercising your way to a more youthful complexion. However, if you choose to have surgery, these exercises do not interfere with or contradict any previous facial surgery or cosmetic treatment. As a matter of fact, the program works very well to help maintain the results you may achieve after such procedures.

Lawrence Birnbaum, M.D., a Beverly Hills plastic surgeon says, "Exercises are extremely beneficial to both pre– and post–operative cosmetic surgery patients. Exercises can also help anyone lift sagging facial skin via building up the fifty-seven facial muscles."

In this book you will be instructed how to isolate and work each of the muscles of the face and neck using advanced techniques.

It will be just as if you had a personal trainer! You will then learn how to massage your face to bring a lasting glow and feeling of revitalization to your skin. This is a thoroughly enjoyable reward after completing the exercise regimen. As you advance, you will fine-tune your appearance safely and effectively. This program can be easily customized to fit your lifestyle and age and takes into account the importance of environmental factors, like how to adjust to seasonal and hormonal changes.

Equally as important is the implementation of an excellent skin-care protocol paired with the nutrition and dietary secrets known to immediately improve the look and feel of your skin. You will learn what skin-care products to use, what foods to eat and when to eat them, and which ones to avoid at all cost. You will also discover some of the most coveted beauty secrets from around the world that have been keeping women looking and feeling their best for centuries. Most are simple and easy for you to replicate at home with a quick trip to your local health food or grocery store.

I wrote this book to share what I have learned: how and why to perform facial exercises and massage techniques. I also wanted to offer a comprehensive guide to healthy approaches to skin-care based on the research and information I have gathered. My hope is that once you have this information in hand, you will begin to make healthier choices, because let's face it— everyone wants to look younger. You just need to know how to achieve that goal without putting yourself at risk. If you can do something that immediately improves your looks while also improving your overall health, then you will truly have something to smile about.

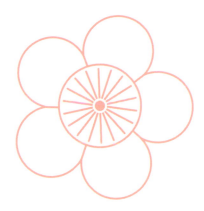

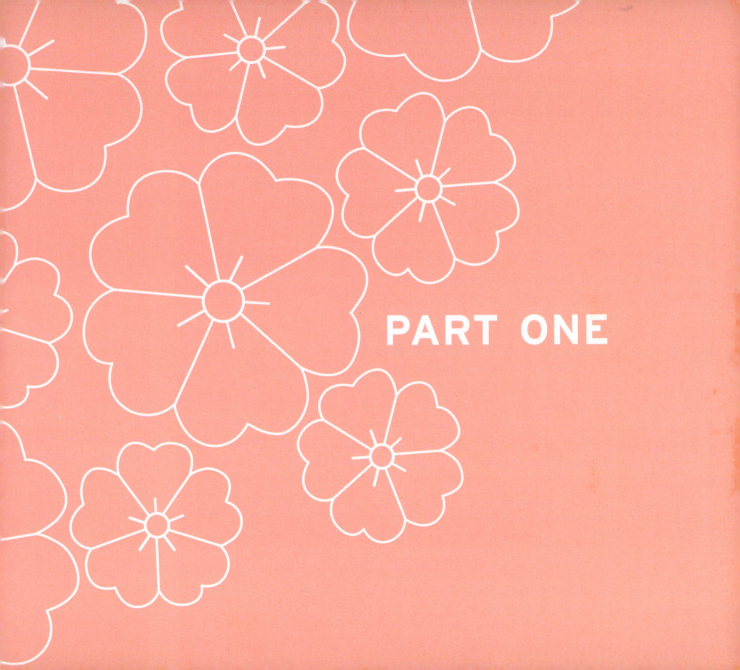

PART ONE

CHAPTER 1

HOW AND WHY THE SKIN AGES

RESEARCH shows that there are two types of aging. Aging caused by the genes you are born with is called intrinsic (internal or chronological) aging, and aging caused by external factors, such as the environment, is referred to as extrinsic aging. Intrinsic aging is a natural process that involves, among other things, the shortening of the life span of your cells. By the time you are an adult, the life span of your cells is less than half of what it was when you were a child. For example, it takes you longer to heal from cuts and scrapes, you begin to bruise more easily, your circulation decreases, and toxins are eliminated at a slower rate. This is the normal aging process, and there's not much we can do to stop it. The factors affecting extrinsic aging, however, can be controlled, so it is these that we will focus on in this chapter.

In your **twenties,** your skin appears firm and virtually wrinkle free. However, within the skin, the production of both collagen and elastin—the substances that enable skin to bounce back from sun expo- sure, wounds, acne, and the like—slows down. This process is accelerated by repeated exposure to the sun's harmful ultraviolet (UV) rays.

This, along with a slight decrease in the ability of dead skin cells to shed, begins the signs of intrinsic aging. Failing to properly protect your skin from the sun's damaging rays at this age (as many people do), and other unhealthy lifestyle choices often made by the young and uninitiated, cause long-term damage and exacerbate the visible signs of aging. Although the signs might not become noticeable until you are well into your thirties, the inevitable process of aging has begun.

In your **thirties,** lines begin to form around the eyes, called crow's feet, between the brows, called glabellar lines, and on the forehead, called transverse lines. Collagen and elastin production continues to slow down, and the skin becomes puffier, espe- cially around the eye area. How you protect, treat, nourish, and strengthen your skin at this age can mean a great deal when it comes to your long-term health and beauty. As you grow older, it will make the difference between looking younger than you are, or, unfortunately, looking much older.

In your **forties,** you can expect to see an even greater loss of elasticity in the skin. The face also begins to lose volume as the skin's fat and collagen begin to diminish. The skin becomes more transparent, the corners of the mouth start to turn down, and age spots may appear or darken. The skin may also become drier due to decreased levels of estrogen.

In your **fifties,** gravity really starts to have an impact. It causes the tip of the nose to droop, the ears to elongate, the eyelids to fall, and the jowls to become more pronounced.

In your **sixties and beyond,** the impact of gravity that you began to see in your fifties becomes even more pronounced. In addition, your face can appear to be puffy and tired all day. Inflammation and fluid build-up are more prevalent at this point, as are fatty deposits under the eyes and chin.

Intrinsic aging is inevitable, however there are ways to help slow the effects of this

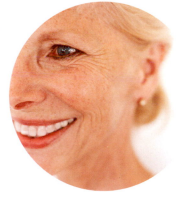

natural process. One of the most important ways to decelerate the aging clock is to make sure you are nourishing your body properly. Good nutrition is essential, but you have to eat what is right for you. Many people suffer from food intolerances and allergies and do not even know it. Oftentimes, unbeknownst to you, the food you most enjoy may be causing digestive problems and headaches, and sapping your energy. You may not see the correlation between what you're eating and how you feel afterwards. If you suffer from any of these symptoms, it's not a bad idea to consult your physician, as well as a nutritionist, and adopt a diet plan that's right for your body.

In addition to proper nutrition, it is essential to get plenty of sleep and drink lots of water, preferably with lemon. As you may know, lemon contains lots of vitamin C and helps reduce inflammation. Try to minimize stress through exercise and massage, and of course, do not smoke!

One of the most important ways to decelerate the aging clock is to make sure you are nourishing your body properly.

Extrinsic aging is responsible for most of the visible signs of prematurely aged skin. One example of this type of aging is prolonged exposure to the sun's harmful UV rays, which is called photoaging. Although it may seem as if these signs appear out of nowhere (often in the form of wrinkles), they have actually been building up under the skin's surface for years. With repeated exposure to the sun, the skin loses the ability to repair itself; thus the damage accumulates. Most skin cancer occurs in prematurely aged skin. Increasing numbers of cases of melanoma (skin cancer) have been well documented in the last few years, perhaps due to the depletion of the ozone. But one thing is for sure: permanent skin damage and disease occur because of accumulated destruction within the skin from previous years of prolonged sun exposure. That is why it is essential for you take steps now to protect not only yourself, but your children as well, from further damage that could lead to skin cancer. By educating your children and applying sunscreen to their skin whenever they are exposed to sunlight for extended amounts of time, you can help protect them from the harmful effects of the sun's burning rays. After just a few instances

"I have been using the Facial Fitness exercises for about a month and a half, and I can see a big difference in my skin. My jawline has tightened quite a bit, the wrinkles on my forehead are almost gone, and my brow area has lifted a little. I am quite happy with the program."

—RITA MOLFETAS

of being sunburned as a child, a person is already at an increased risk of developing skin cancer later in life.

The scientific details of how and why the sun damages your skin are very technical, but suffice it to say that it's essential to protect your skin as much as possible if you want to avoid skin cancer and premature aging. A few ways to ensure that you are being protected from the sun's harmful rays are to wear protective clothing, including a hat and sunglasses, and use sunscreen on a daily basis—no matter what time of year or in what climate. Many excellent skin-care lines now contain a broad-spectrum sunscreen with an SPF (sun protection factor) of fifteen or higher in their day-creams, so it is very simple to protect your skin as you moisturize. Make sure that the products you apply contain both UVA and UVB protec-

tion, and apply a moisturizer with sunblock liberally, letting it dry completely before applying your makeup or putting on clothing.

After just a few instances of being sunburned as a child, a person is already at an increased risk of developing skin cancer later in life.

In addition to the sun, the skin has many more enemies. Among them are smoking, excess alcohol consumption, crash dieting, dehydration, exposure to chemicals contained in some cosmetics and skin-care products, pollution, and stress, just to name a few. Each of these, in its own sinister way, damages the skin. Some cause deterioration of collagen and elastin, others may interfere with the rate at which new cells turn over. This kind of damage dramatically affects the skin's tone and outer appearance. Because of this, fine lines, wrinkles, and skin discoloration begin to occur, and skin begins to age prematurely.

It is essential to minimize exposure to those sources of skin damage mentioned above by taking preventative steps to ensure as little damage to the skin as possible. No one wants to accelerate the aging process, but unfortunately an unhealthy lifestyle does just that.

As you learn to avoid these potentially harmful factors and begin a healthy routine of skin-care, it is vital to add a facial exercise and massage program to your daily regimen

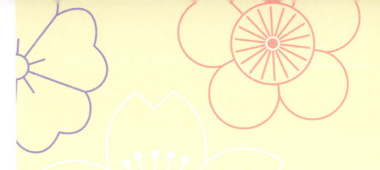

"This is the greatest thing I've done for my appearance yet. The results I've seen after just a few weeks are remarkably noticeable, and it was so easy. I highly recommend it to anyone looking for a safe, effective alternative to surgery."

—LINDA CONNOLLY

so that you don't neglect the muscles of the face and neck. Simply moving your face by making various expressions or eating does not mean all the muscles are being worked and strengthened effectively. Consistently exercising and massaging the facial muscles properly will ensure a more youthful and toned appearance for years to come.

Exercise and massage are intrinsic parts of a healthy lifestyle, so why not have your face benefit as well?

Through exercise and massage, the muscles become toned and circulation increases, thus allowing the waste products and toxins trapped within the skin's layers to be eliminated more efficiently. Exercise also helps stimulate the skin, giving it a youthful glow. The massage program alone provides both immediate and long-term benefits, not the least of which is a reduction in stress, but when used in conjunction with the facial exercises, a healthy, firm foundation is formed on which to build and maintain youthful-looking skin.

By following the Facial Fitness program and adopting a proactive skin-care regimen, you will be able to actually reverse many of the visible signs of aging by protecting, strengthening, and toning the facial muscles. Your cheeks will seem less hollow, the corners of your mouth will be lifted, your eyes will widen, your neck will become smoother, and your jowls will begin to lift.

As you know, a healthy lifestyle, good nutrition, and plenty of rest will greatly improve your overall health. Exercise and massage are intrinsic parts of a healthy lifestyle, so why not have your face benefit as well? So much about the way you feel is projected on your face. When someone is truly healthy in mind and body you can see it immediately. She or he exudes confidence and well-being, which is very attractive to others. It's quite simple—when you look good, you feel good. The Facial Fitness program is an all-natural way to promote a healthy, youthful appearance. Follow the program carefully, and in no time you will begin to see amazing results right before your eyes. Your facial features will become more defined, and you will be able to sculpt your face as you would your body, through the use of specific exercises designed to enhance your own natural beauty.

"I can't believe the results I experienced after just two weeks of using the Facial Fitness system. My jawline is tighter and the lines around my eyes have just about vanished. It's incredible!"

—GRACE SURDIS

CHAPTER 2

THE BENEFITS OF FACIAL EXERCISE AND MASSAGE

FACIAL EXERCISE AND MASSAGE have many benefits. Not only will they tone and tighten the muscles of the face and neck, but they will instantly rejuvenate tired looking skin by increasing the blood flow and circulation, revitalizing the skin's surface with a flushed, healthy glow. The exercises are great to do as a quick pick-me-up whenever you want to look rested and refreshed, and you will see the long-term benefits of reduced wrinkles and an overall younger look in no time.

Here is what you will achieve by following the Facial Fitness program:

- A youthful, healthy appearance

- The appearance of a longer neck through proper posture

- An evenly balanced head by strengthening the neck muscles

- A clear, radiant complexion by helping to release toxins from the skin and increase circulation

- A relaxed forehead by training the muscles to be at ease

- Uplifted eyes by strengthening the muscles above the eyes

- Raised eyebrows through toning the muscles above the brow

- Firmer cheeks by strengthening the facial and jaw muscles

- Upturned corners of the mouth by toning the nasal-labial muscles

- Fuller, smoother lips by toning and relaxing the muscles around the mouth

- A well-shaped nose by toning the nasal muscles and thinning the appearance of the nose

- A well-shaped jawline by lifting the muscles of the face and neck

- Increased awareness of your facial expressions through a conscious effort to visualize each and every muscle as it is being trained and strengthened

- Better control of your facial expressions as you become aware of the facial muscles and how they react when a particular emotion is portrayed

- ❧ Alleviated symptoms of TMJ disorder by strengthening the muscles and ligaments and encouraging increased circulation to the affected area

- ❧ Alleviated symptoms of Bell's palsy by strengthening the affected muscles or group of muscles and learning to relax them

Not only does the Facial Fitness program help maintain a youthful appearance, but it can relieve painful facial conditions. For years, specialized physical therapists and physicians have been prescribing facial exercises as part of a rehabilitation regimen for the treatment of conditions such as TMJ disorder and Bell's palsy. Facial resistance training is now being offered at many rehabilitation facilities to address these conditions. Studies showing their effectiveness are readily available online.

Bell's palsy is a sudden and debilitating condition that is a type of paralysis or weakness of the muscles in the face, thought to be due to inflammation of the seventh cranial nerve, also known as the facial nerve. Gaye Cronin, OTD, OTR, the director of the Neuromuscular Facial Retraining Program at the Atlanta Ear Clinic, says, "Loss of facial function can affect a person's quality of life, self-esteem, oral motor controls, and eyelid function. Other problems can develop as well, such as abnormal movement patterns, abnormal tone, eye irritations, and taste or chewing problems." Bell's palsy can be effectively treated by performing targeted facial exercises. Of course, you should always consult your doctor before performing any exercise regimen, especially one designed to relieve a particular condition. Todd Henkelmann, PT, MS, of the University of Pittsburgh Medical Center Facial Nerve Center, says that those suffering from acute cases of Bell's palsy should not perform exercises during the first few weeks of the syndrome, due to flaccidity of the affected side.

Through the use of facial neuromuscular training, strength and stability can be restored to the affected area of the face. Authorities on Bell's palsy recommend that patients familiarize themselves with the muscles of the face and neck to help isolate the muscle action, and they also suggest performing the exercises in front of a mirror to ensure that they are being done properly and effectively. Additionally, many authorities recommend massage as part of the routine in all stages of recovery.

Gaye Cronin adds that, "Neuromuscular facial retraining programs have proven to be successful in the recovery of facial function. Facial exercises for specific, isolated movements are included in these programs." The following are examples of functional facial exercises created by Cronin to help alleviate symptoms of Bell's palsy. If you suffer from Bell's palsy, practice these exercises once a day, in addition to my recommended exercises later in the book.

When rehabilitation is the goal, remember to work the muscles gently as you progress through your routine and do not overwork any one area.

To increase eyelid closure: Hold a target approximately 25 degrees below eye level. Keep your eyes on the target and slowly lower your eyelids. Try not to allow your eyeballs to roll up or out. Try to keep the target in focus until the lids completely close.

To increase lip closure: Face a mirror and press your lips together. Hold for 5 counts, then move your lips into a pucker position and hold for 5 counts. Try to keep your lips centered and do not allow them to pull toward the stronger side.

To decrease synkinesis (abnormal movement patterns): Face a mirror and make small puckers with your mouth. As soon as you see or feel your eyelid muscles pull or squint, stop the mouth movement. Make a conscious effort to isolate the mouth movements from the eye movements.

When rehabilitation is the goal, remember to work the muscles gently as you progress through your routine, and do not overwork any one area. Symmetry and balance, as well as regained movement, are the goals when exercising for medical reasons, so do not overdo it. Exercise in short sessions and stop when you begin to feel fatigued. Exercises and massage techniques recommended specifically for the rehabilitation of Bell's palsy are discussed later in the book.

Temporomandibular joint disorder, or TMJ disorder, is another common condition affecting millions of people. This extremely painful disorder stems from an unwanted deviation of the jaw when the patient opens his or her mouth. TMJ disorder usually occurs when the teeth are misaligned or a person suffers an injury, such as a blow to the face, or an indirect trauma, such as whiplash, which causes a displacement of the cartilage where the jaw is attached to the skull. This displacement in turn causes a painful sense of pressure and stretching of the associated sensory nerves. Another condition known as bruxism, which is an abnormal grinding of the teeth, is also a leading cause of TMJ disorder. Bruxism is usually accompanied by a popping or clicking of the jaw, as well as sharp, sudden pain, which may radiate up and across the face.

Facial exercises are used to help re-educate the jaw to open correctly, thus alleviating many of these symptoms. According to Dr. Richard H. Keller, DDS,

of the American Academy of Biomechanical Trauma and Cranio-Facial Pain, "Facial exercises, especially for the muscles of mastication and those involving the tongue, are very effective in the realignment of the jaw and help to alleviate the pressure and pain associated with TMJ disorder. Approximately 85 percent of the patients using these exercises, often called neuro-muscular reeducation, experience success. Others may need further treatment, such as injections known as neuraltherapy and/or the use of a splint to further alleviate pain and correct any misalignment."

The Facial Fitness program was originated with TMJ disorders in mind and has been proven effective in alleviating many of the symptoms associated with it when the exercises and massage techniques are performed on a consistent basis. You'll find specific exercises and massage techniques for the rehabilitation of TMJ disorder later in the book.

As with any exercise program, consistency is the key to success, so make the Facial Fitness program part of your everyday routine, whether your goal is rehabilitation or just simple toning. Before long you will begin to see and feel results.

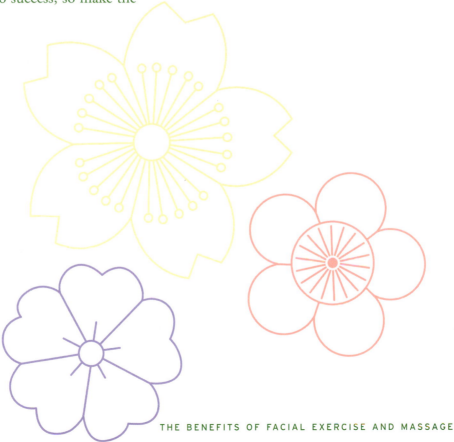

CHAPTER 3

THE MUSCLES AND HOW THEY WORK

ON THE FOLLOWING PAGES are diagrams of the head, face, and neck muscles. As you will see, they form a complex and intricate system that works synergistically to provide form and function, as well as to express emotion. Like all our muscles, if they are left static, they begin to slacken over time, creating the appearance of tired, aged, unhealthy skin. For example, when your face is at rest while you are reading, sleeping, driving, watching television, working on the computer, or listening intently, it is generally motionless. Unless you are making some involuntary movements such as pursing your lips or squinting, the muscles on your face are, for the most part, not engaged.

Once you become aware of the way you look when you are occupied with a specific task or deep in thought, you can begin to train your "facial posture."

Have you ever unexpectedly caught a glimpse of yourself in a mirror? Were you surprised to see the expression you were making? Most of the time we are not aware of what we truly look like. Once you become aware of the way you look when you are occupied with a specific task or deep in thought, you can begin to train your "facial posture." Much like becoming aware of your body's posture and straightening up when you slouch, you should become aware of your facial posture and do the same. Incorporating a facial exercise routine into your everyday life is a terrific way to tone and tighten these muscles.

Actors are often taught to become acutely aware of their facial expressions and some are even trained to perform facial exercises to make themselves fully conscious of each expression they're making. Having command of these muscles helps actors convey to the audience the emotions they intend to project so that their characters are believable and convincing.

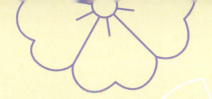

"I am a method actor in New York who has been using facial exercises for years without even knowing it. In the method I use, it is a process of complete body relaxation. The theory is that the more relaxed you are the easier it is to draw on a sense memory for whatever role you are playing. When I first started taking acting classes, my instructor showed us facial exercises to get in touch with the muscles in the face. When you are in tune with your muscles and aware of any stress you may be holding in these muscles, it becomes easier to relax them. The instructors informed us that one of the by-products of these exercises would be a more youthful appearance. Being an actor approaching forty years old, this can come in pretty handy. When one of my friends told me about the Facial Fitness program, I was very excited and had to check it out. The first time I watched the DVD, I was hooked. For years I have been struggling with the muscles in my forehead. I could never seem to relax them, which has given me wrinkles. Not only has the Facial Fitness program brought me more in tune with these muscles, but my wrinkles are starting to go away."

—GEORGE NETZ

Listed from top to bottom are the major muscles of the head, face, and neck and a brief description of their function. Diagrams of the muscles can be found on pages 45 to 47.

MUSCLES OF THE SCALP

The *galea aponeurotica* is a flat tendon that covers the top part of the cranium and connects the *frontalis* and the *occipitalis* muscles.

The *occipitalis* is a small muscle located at the back of the head. It is part of the muscle group that moves the scalp.

The *frontalis* is the muscle that covers the forehead. In conjunction with the *corrugator*, it is responsible for raising and lowering the scalp, forehead, eyebrows, and the top of the nose. Constantly raising and lowering the eyebrows through expression causes deep horizontal lines across the forehead. Toning these muscles properly will help to smooth out these lines, and make you more aware of your facial expressions.

MUSCLES OF THE EYE

There are several muscles in the eye area. The *orbicularis oculi* is primarily responsible for the opening and closing of the eye, and the *procerus* is responsible for the movement of the skin between the eyebrows.

The *levator palpebrae,* the muscle found behind the *orbicularis oculi* in the upper eyelid, is also responsible for the opening and closing of the eye.

Strengthening these muscles will help to fight the gravitational pull on these delicate areas of the face. Squinting causes many of the lines and wrinkles that surround the eyes and betray your age. You can diminish the signs of aging caused by sun exposure by protecting your eyes from the sun by wearing sunblock and sunglasses.

MUSCLES OF THE NOSE

Yes, even the nose has muscles. Try flaring your nostrils and you will feel the anterior and posterior *dilatator* muscles working to increase the airflow through the nose.

The *nasalis,* which is located over the bridge of the nose, helps compress the nostrils, as does the *depressor septi.* Strengthening these muscles will help reshape the nose and prevent the tip from drooping.

MUSCLES OF THE MOUTH

The muscles responsible for opening and closing the mouth are known as the *orbicularis oris* and the *caninus.* These muscles completely surround the mouth and are connected to the nose, cheeks, lips, and chin.

The *mentalis* is located on the front of the chin. It raises and lowers the chin and lower lip. The *quadratus labii superioris* lies above the top lip and the *quadratus labii inferioris* lies below the lower lip.

MUSCLES OF MASTICATION

The muscles of mastication—including the *pterygoideus internus,* the *pterygoideus externus,* the *masseter,* the *temporalis,* and the *buccinator*—work together to give the jaw the ability to operate in all of its vital functions, such as opening and closing the mouth, chewing, grinding, yawning, and, of course, speaking. Toning these muscles helps alleviate the appearance of facial drooping and can relieve the painful symptoms of TMJ disorder.

MUSCLES OF THE NECK

Known as the *platysma* muscles, the muscles of the neck run from the corners of the mouth to the jaw, and down to the collarbone in the front of the neck on either side. They assist in the operation of the jaw and help with swallowing. As you age, these muscles start to separate, causing the appearance of cords running down either side of the neck, sometimes with loose skin in between. The *sternocleidomastoid* is primarily responsible for turning the head from side to side, and along with the *trapezesius* muscle, allows you to partially rotate the head, as well as move it up and down.

Now that you are familiar with these major muscles of the face and neck, you will be able to focus on them as you isolate a particular muscle or group of muscles and visualize them as you tone and strengthen them through the Facial Fitness program.

There's no time like the present, so let's get you started on your way to a more youthful, healthy, and dynamic appearance. Remember: repetition is essential to your success, so stick with it, and in no time you will begin to see results. This remarkable method of strengthening will give a natural lift to your face and neck—and take years off your appearance.

MUSCLES OF THE HEAD, FACE, AND NECK
(FRONTAL VIEW)

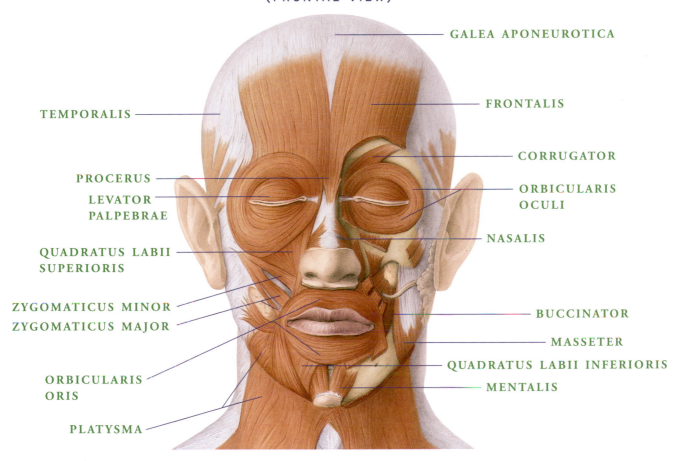

GALEA APONEUROTICA

FRONTALIS

CORRUGATOR

TEMPORALIS

ORBICULARIS
OCULI

PROCERUS

LEVATOR
PALPEBRAE

NASALIS

QUADRATUS LABII
SUPERIORIS

ZYGOMATICUS MINOR

ZYGOMATICUS MAJOR

BUCCINATOR

MASSETER

QUADRATUS LABII INFERIORIS

ORBICULARIS
ORIS

MENTALIS

PLATYSMA

INTERNAL MUSCLES OF THE JAW
(SIDE VIEW)

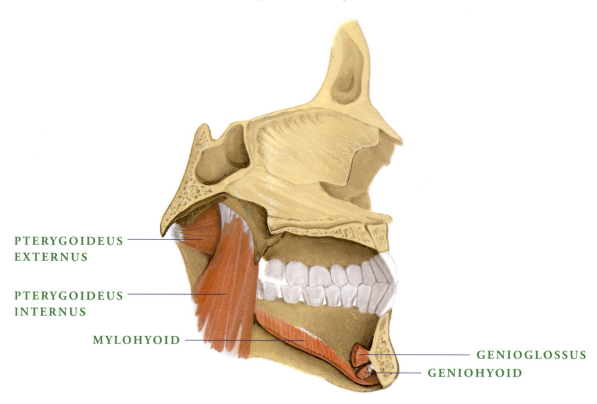

PTERYGOIDEUS
EXTERNUS

PTERYGOIDEUS
INTERNUS

MYLOHYOID

GENIOGLOSSUS

GENIOHYOID

MUSCLES OF THE HEAD, FACE, AND NECK
(SIDE VIEW)

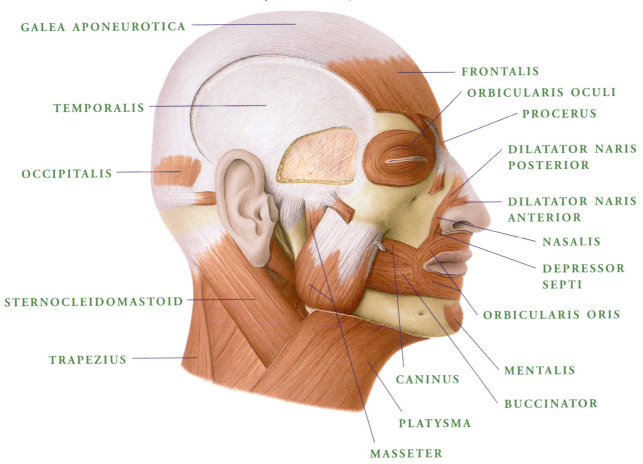

GALEA APONEUROTICA

TEMPORALIS

OCCIPITALIS

STERNOCLEIDOMASTOID

TRAPEZIUS

FRONTALIS

ORBICULARIS OCULI

PROCERUS

DILATATOR NARIS POSTERIOR

DILATATOR NARIS ANTERIOR

NASALIS

DEPRESSOR SEPTI

ORBICULARIS ORIS

MENTALIS

BUCCINATOR

PLATYSMA

MASSETER

CANINUS

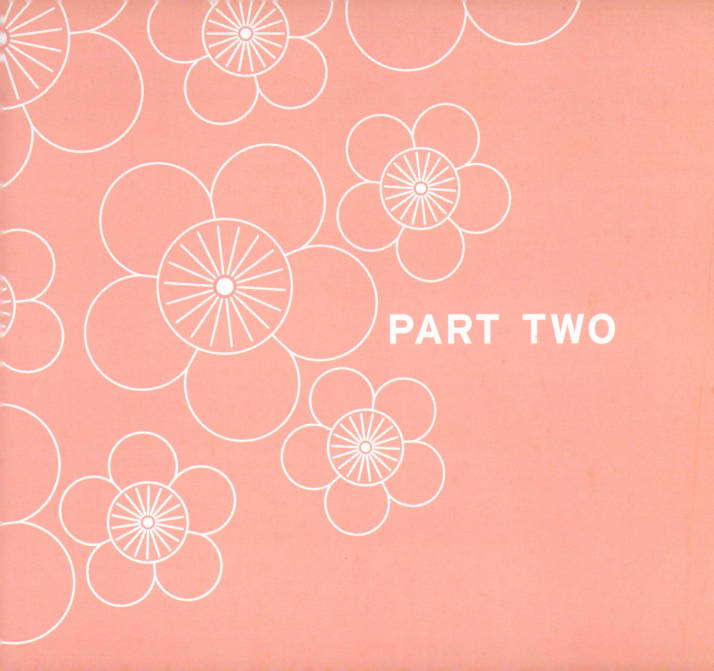

PART TWO

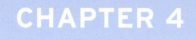

CHAPTER 4

THE EXERCISES

WHEN YOU FIRST BEGIN the Facial Fitness program, I recommend that you perform the exercises and massage techniques in front of a mirror to ensure proper hand placement, and to make sure that you are doing them correctly. It is also advisable for you to begin by doing them in the morning or in the evening when your face is freshly cleansed and you are in a relaxed state. Try to dedicate at least fifteen minutes to your facial exercise program at first, and soon you will become so familiar with the techniques that you will be able to perform them anywhere, anytime.

You may find that you are holding your breath while doing the exercises. That is fine for the ten-second duration of each exercise, but make sure to take a deep, cleansing breath when you complete the exercise, and remember to breathe normally between each set.

You should feel the muscles begin to fatigue, or "burn." This is a good sign. It means you are working effectively.

Before you begin, make sure your hands are thoroughly washed and, if possible, apply moisturizer to your face to help prevent unnecessary stretching of the facial skin.

The Facial Fitness program consists of twelve basic exercises designed to work many of the fifty-seven muscles of the face and neck synergistically, creating a stronger and more toned appearance. Once you have achieved the initial benefits of the Facial Fitness program, you will be ready to move on to the more advanced techniques to further sculpt and enhance your youthful look.

These techniques can be added to your daily facial exercise routine gradually, and you may increase the hold duration and number of repetitions to advance your workout even further. You should feel the muscles begin to fatigue, or "burn." This is a good sign. It means you are working effectively. (If you are using these exercises for rehabilitative purposes, however, you should stop before you feel the muscle fatigue.) Remember to relax and breathe normally between each set.

When you finish the Facial Fitness routine, you should feel completely relaxed and your skin will look rested and rejuvenated immediately. Repeat these facial exercises once a day for the first three weeks, then every other day to maintain your toned and youthful appearance.

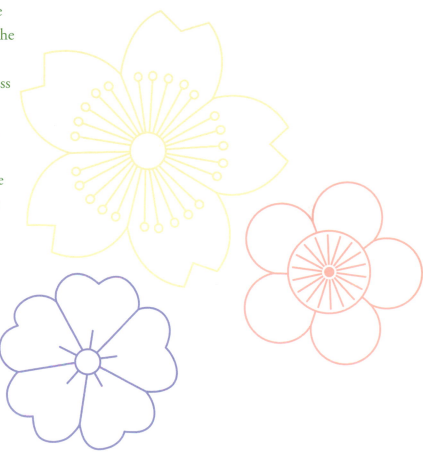

THE BASIC EXERCISES

THE ADVANCED EXERCISES

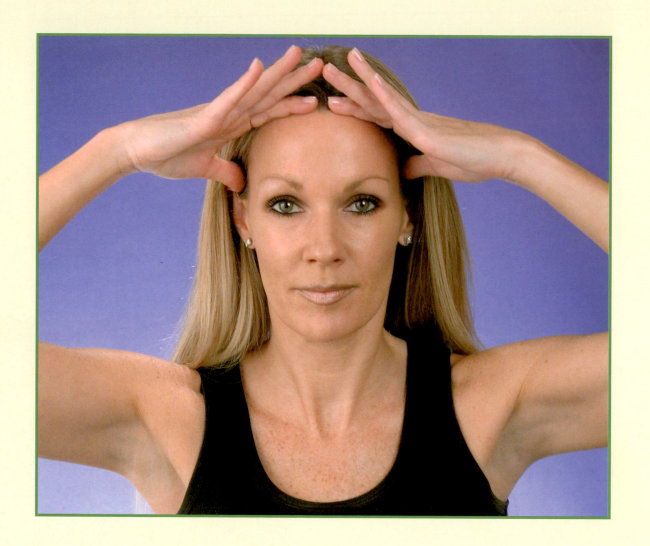

THE FOREHEAD LIFT

This exercise works the *galea aponeurotica*, *frontalis*, and *corrugator* muscles to help diminish horizontal lines on the forehead.

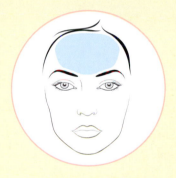

Place your index fingers flat along your hairline. While pushing up with your index fingers, push down with your eyebrows. Hold down for 10 seconds. Repeat 3 times, each time to the count of 10.

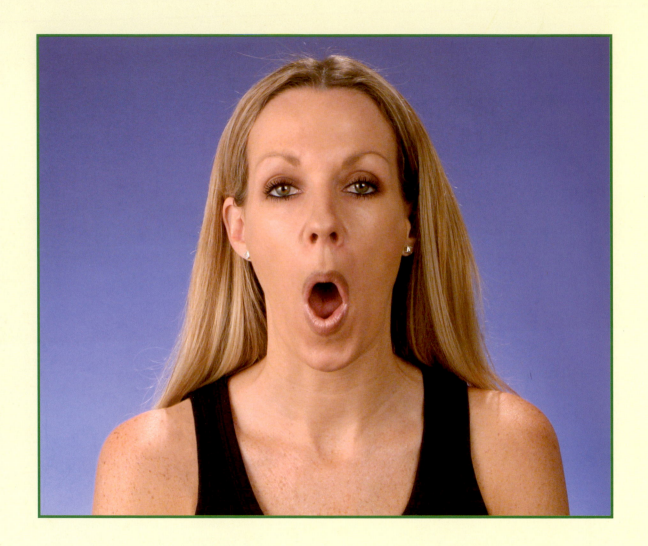

THE NASAL-LABIAL LINE DIMINISHER

This exercise works the muscles surrounding the nose
and mouth called the *orbicularis oris* and the *caninus,* and is designed
to help diminish the lines on either side of the mouth, referred to
as the nasal-labial lines, or marionette lines.

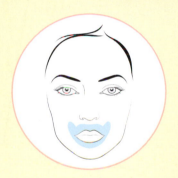

Open your mouth wide, making your face very long.
With your mouth open, slowly say, "ooh, ooh, ooh, ooh"
10 times. By vocalizing this sound, you will make the muscles
surrounding the mouth contract and relax, thereby
strengthening the surrounding muscles.

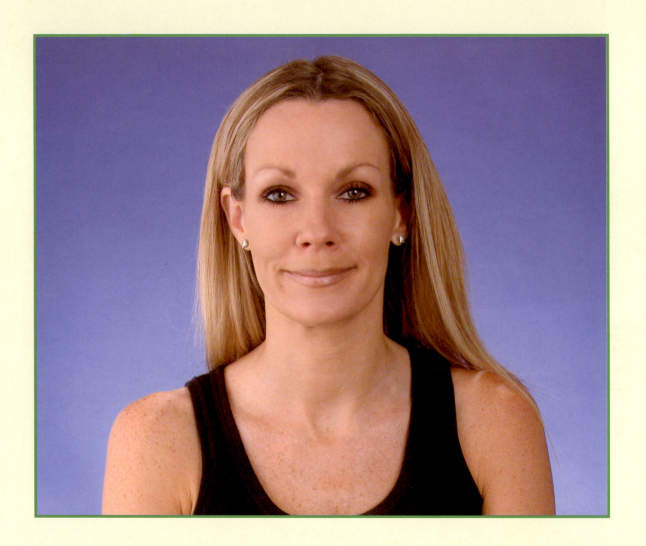

THE NOSE THINNER

Did you know that your nose and ears continue to grow throughout
your life because of the cartilage they contain? After all, W.C. Fields wasn't
born with that nose. This exercise will strengthen the muscles
that run across and alongside the nose, called the *nasalis,* the *procerus,* and
the *depressor septi,* and will help keep your nose looking long and slim.

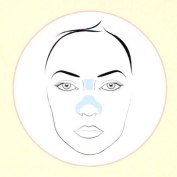

Push the tip of your nose down and
flare your nostrils for 10 seconds. Repeat 3 times,
each time to the count of 10.

This exercise is recommended for the treatment of Bell's palsy.

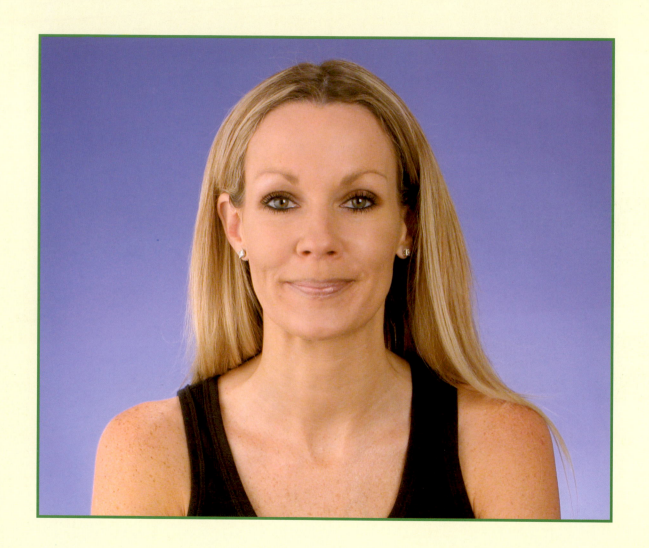

FACIAL FITNESS

THE MOUTH LIFTER

This exercise will tone and train the muscles near the corners of the mouth to lift, creating a more youthful appearance. The muscles affected are the *orbicularis oris,* the *quadratus labii superioris,* the *quadratus labii inferioris,* and the *caninus.*

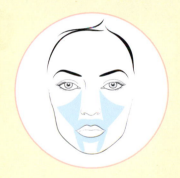

Tighten the corners of your mouth very hard and pull your lips together. Hold for 10 seconds. Repeat 3 times, each time to the count of 10.

This exercise is recommended for the treatment of Bell's palsy.

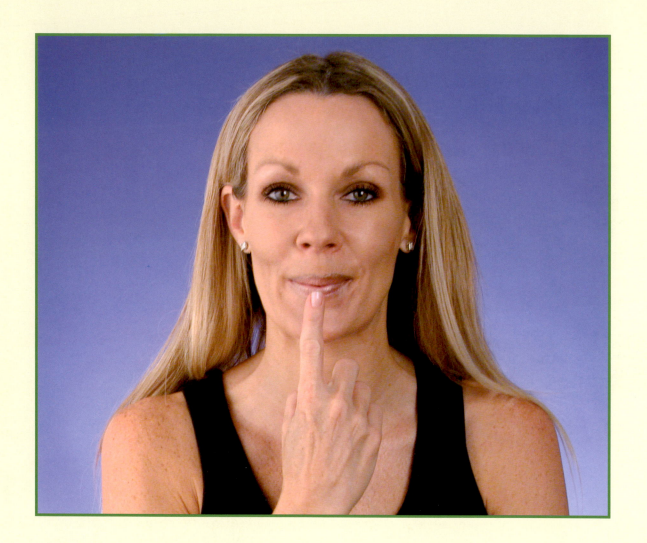

THE LIP PUMPER

This exercise will help increase blood flow to the lips
and the surrounding muscles, known as the *orbicularis oris* and
the *mentalis,* to create a more full and pouty appearance.

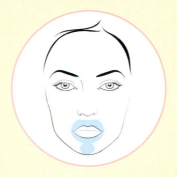

Hold your mouth in a hard pout and try to smile.
While holding this position, try to force a small stream
of air out, just at the center of your lips. Hold your
finger in front of your lips to ensure that the air stream
is thin and steady. Hold for 10 seconds and then relax
and breathe normally. Repeat 3 times,
each time to the count of 10.

This exercise is recommended for the treatment of Bell's palsy.

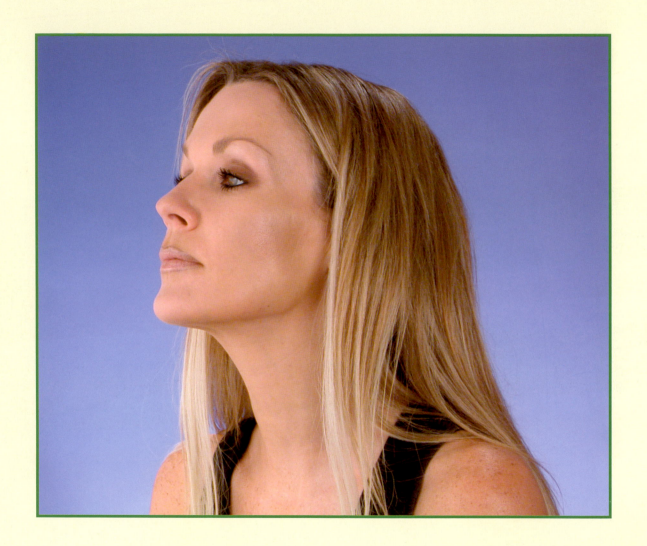

THE NECK STRENGTHENER

This exercise strengthens the muscles in both the front and back of your neck, known as the *platysma,* the *sternocleidomastoid,* and the *trapezius* muscles. This exercise may also be done while lying down on your back.

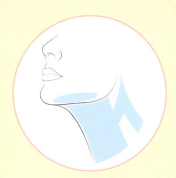

Move your head forward, leading with your bottom jaw. Extend your neck as far forward as you can and hold that position for 10 seconds. Then return to the original position. Repeat this exercise 3 times, holding each extension for 10 seconds.

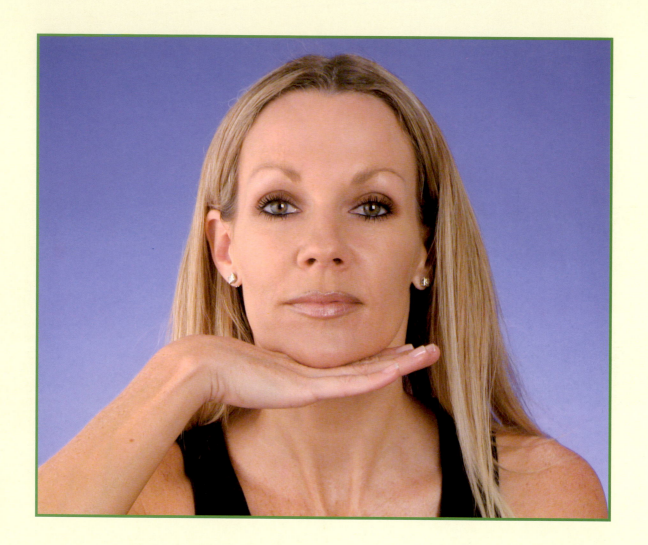

THE JAWLINE ENHANCER

This exercise works the muscles surrounding the jaw—
called the *masseter,* the *pterygoideus internus* and *externus,* the *temporalis,*
and the *buccinator*—as well as the muscles under the chin, such as
the *platysma,* helping to tone and tighten this delicate area.

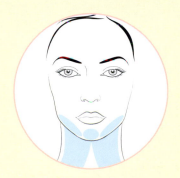

Place your hand palm side down under your chin.
While holding your hand steady for resistance,
push your chin down against your hand 10 times.
Do 3 sets of 10 and then relax.

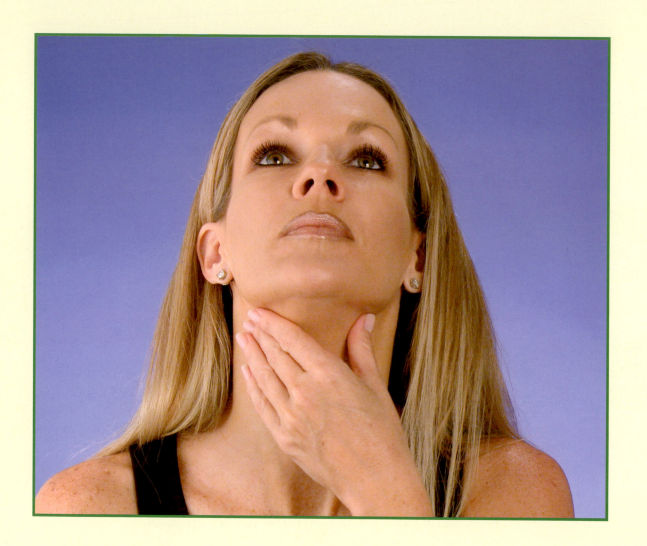

FACIAL FITNESS

THE NECK AND JAWLINE TONER

This technique tones and tightens the *platysma* muscles,
located at the front of the neck as well as on the sides. It also
helps tone the muscles that support the jawline.

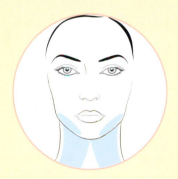

Tilt your head back, extending your bottom jaw.
Feel that your neck is tightened up and hold for 10 seconds.
Repeat 3 times, each time to the count of 10.

This exercise is recommended for the treatment of TMJ disorder.

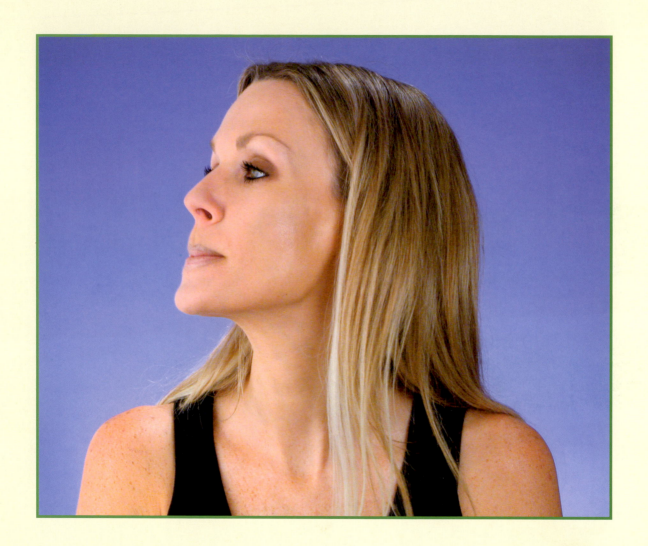

THE NECK AND JAWLINE ENHANCER

Again, this technique is designed to tone the *platysma* muscle
and other muscles along the jawline, helping to prevent
a double chin as well as the appearance of jowls.

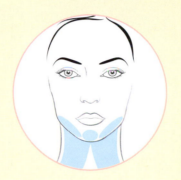

Turn your head to the right, extend your jaw,
and hold for 10 seconds. Return your head back to center.
Now turn your head to the left, extend your jaw,
and hold for 10 seconds. Repeat this exercise 3 times
on each side, each time to the count of 10.

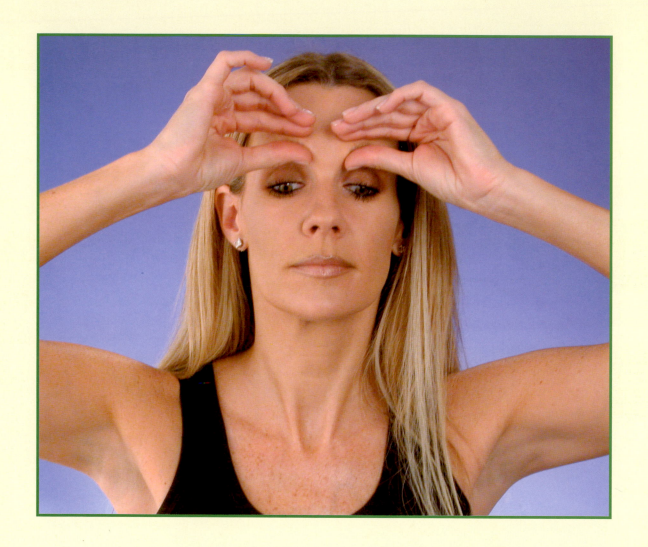

THE VERTICAL LINE DIMINISHER

This exercise is designed to flatten and relax the muscles that
you use when you frown, such as the *frontalis* and the *procerus* muscles,
and to minimize the appearance of deep vertical lines.

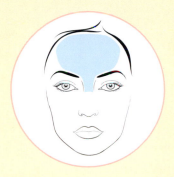

Gently grasp the skin on either side of your face,
just above your nose and between your eyebrows where vertical
lines tend to form. Pull gently in an outward direction
while pushing down with the inside corners of your eyebrows.
Hold for 10 seconds. Repeat 3 times, each time
to the count of 10.

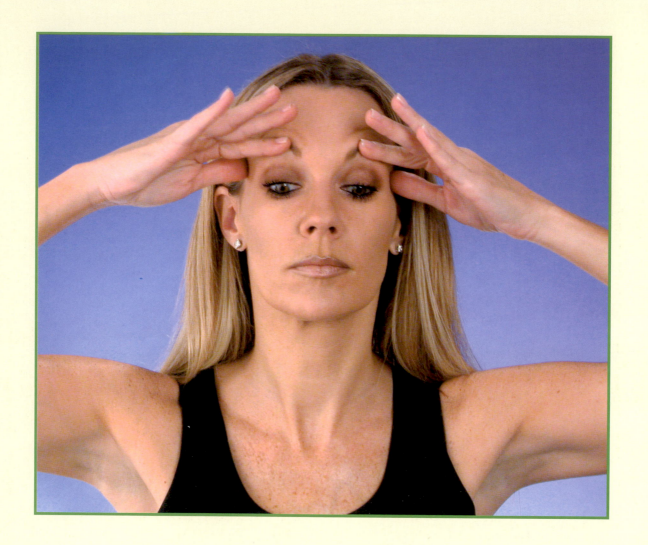

THE TOP EYELID LIFTER

Similar in technique to the Forehead Lift, this exercise is designed to strengthen the upper eyelid muscle, known as the *levator palpebrae,* by opening up the eye and lifting the brow.

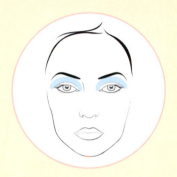

Place your index fingers flat under your eyebrows. Gently push up with your fingers while pushing down with both eyebrows. Hold to the count of 10. Repeat 3 times, each time to the count of 10.

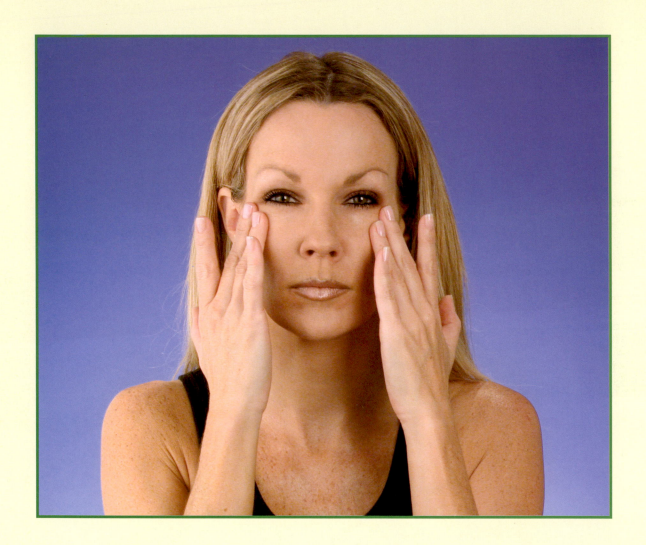

THE UNDER-EYE LINE DIMINISHER

Designed to strengthen the muscles below and around the eyes, known as the *orbicularis oculi,* this technique is essential to reducing puffiness, and it also diminishes the lines that form around the delicate eye area.

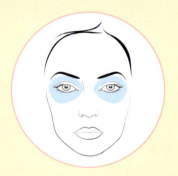

Gently place your middle and ring fingers at the outside corners of your eyes. Squinting with the lower eye muscles, squeeze and release 10 times. Repeat this exercise 3 times, squeezing and releasing 10 times each.

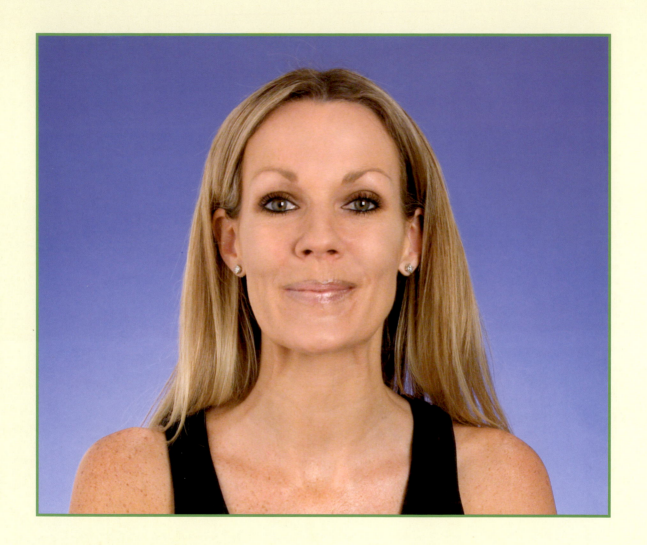

ADVANCED JAWLINE TONERS

These techniques further strengthen the *platysma* muscle under
the chin and along the jawline, as well as the *masseter*.

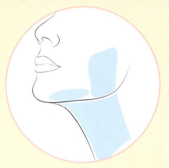

EXERCISE #1

Depress your tongue firmly against the roof of your
mouth, tilt your head back slightly, and hold this position
for 10 seconds. Repeat 3 times, each time to the count of 10.

This exercise is recommended for the treatment of TMJ disorder.

EXERCISE #2

Pull your cheeks back towards your ears (using only your
facial muscles). Feel the ears lift and hold this position
for 10 seconds. Repeat 3 times, each time to the count of 10.

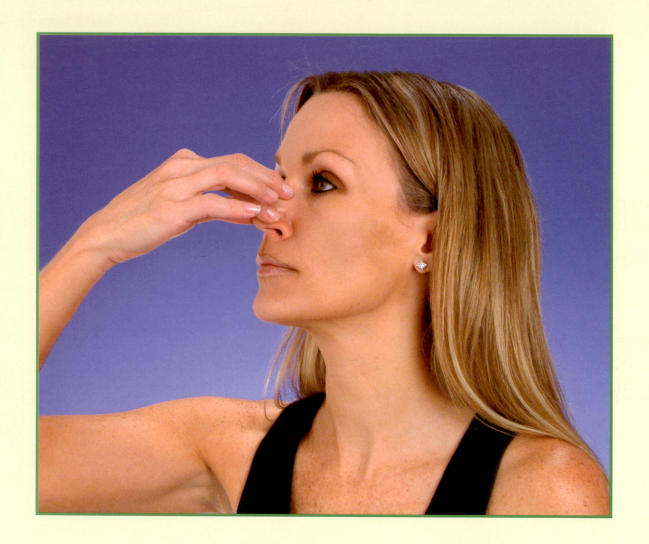

FACIAL FITNESS

THE NOSE DEFINER

This technique will define the nose even more by strengthening the *nasalis* and *depressor septi.*

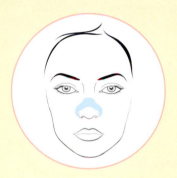

Hold the tip of your nose slightly with your thumb and index finger. Don't squeeze too hard, you want to be able to feel the nostrils flare 10 times and relax. Do 3 sets, flaring your nostrils 10 times for each set.

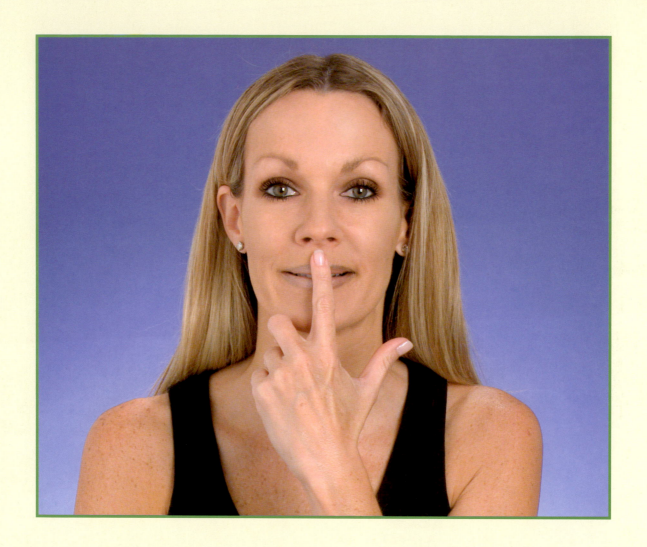

THE UPPER LIP
LINE ERASER

By further toning the *mentalis* muscle, the vertical lines
on the upper lip will begin to diminish.

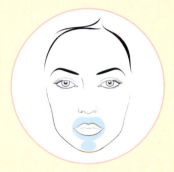

Press your index finger against the cleft
between your lip and nose. Smile with your mouth
slightly ajar and hold for 10 seconds.
Repeat 3 times, each time to the count of 10.

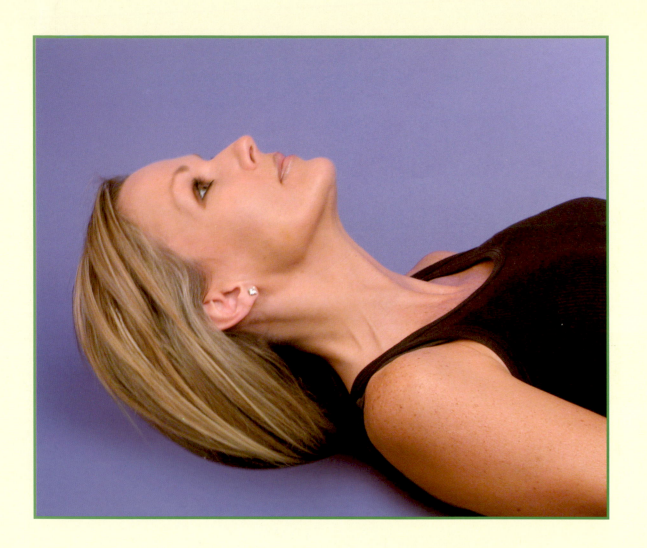

FACIAL FITNESS

HEAD LIFTS FOR DOUBLE CHIN

This exercise helps increase the strength
and stability of both the front and the back of the neck
and tightens the *platysma* muscles.

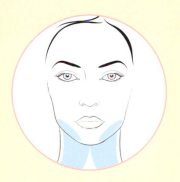

Lie down on your back on the floor.
Lift your head straight up, leading with your chin.
Hold for 3 seconds, then relax. Repeat this 10 times
and relax. You may do as many as 3 sets of 10,
but work up to this gradually to avoid neck strain.

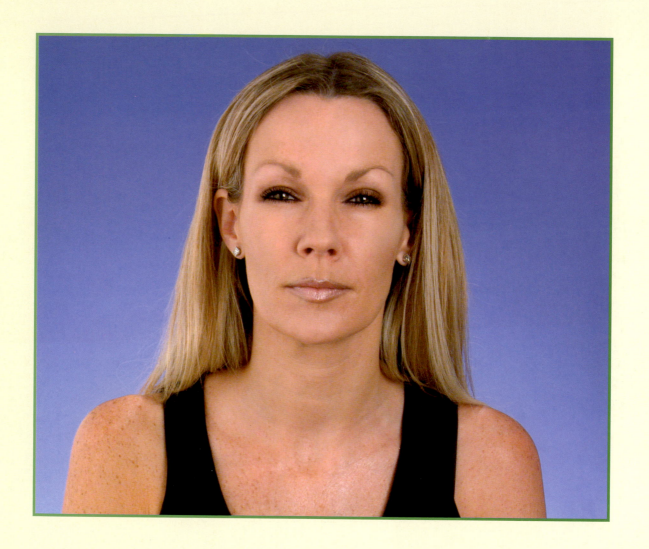

FACIAL FITNESS

THE EYE TONER

This technique is designed to further strengthen
the *orbicularis oculi,* and to diminish the appearance of fine lines
and wrinkles around the eyes.

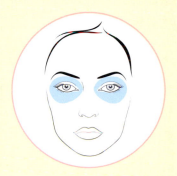

Pull the innermost corners of your eyes up
and hold for 2 seconds. Repeat 10 times and relax.
You may do as many as 3 sets of 10 repetitions.

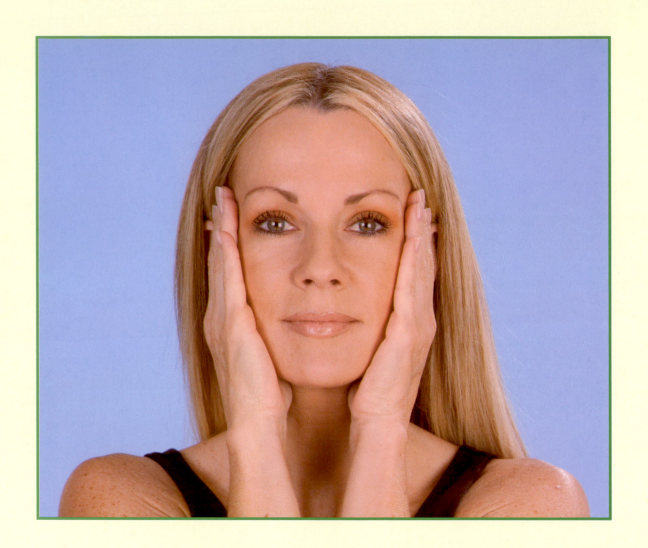

THE FACE LIFTER

This exercise helps to lift and tone the entire face instantly,
by toning the *platysma*, *zygomaticus minor* and *major*,
quadratus labii, and *massater* muscles.

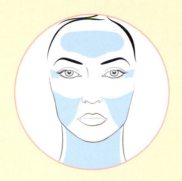

Place your hands on either side of your face and cradle it
in your hands. Lift your entire face using the cheek and neck
muscles by smiling very hard and raising your brows and
forehead. Visualize your entire face moving upward and feel
your face lift within your hands. Hold for 10 seconds
and relax. Repeat 3 times.

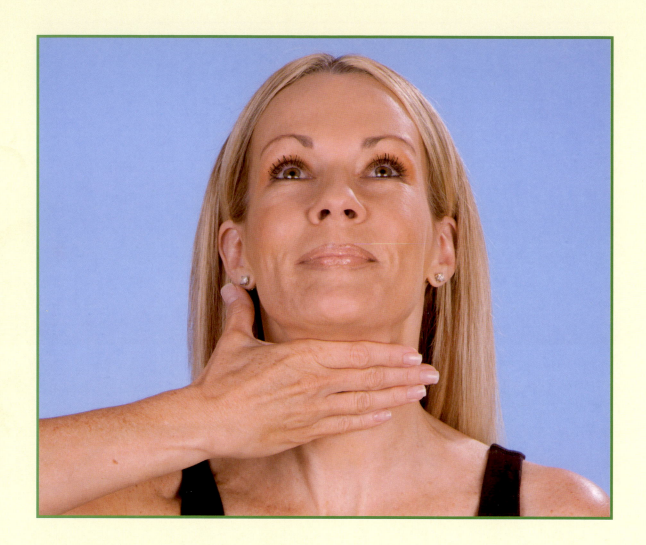

FACIAL FITNESS

THE UNDER-CHIN NECK TIGHTENER

This exercise lifts the neck upward and inward, eliminating banding
around the neck and double chin by reducing the fat deposits under the chin.
It tones the *platysma* and *mentalis* muscles.

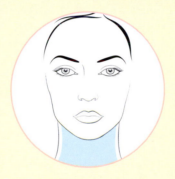

Smile, tilt your head back, and lay your hand across the front of
your neck. Flex the muscles in the front of your neck upward in
a pumping motion 10 times and relax. Repeat 3 times.

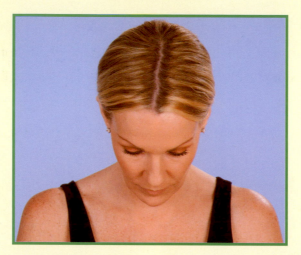

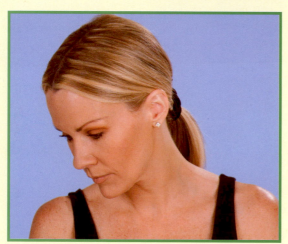

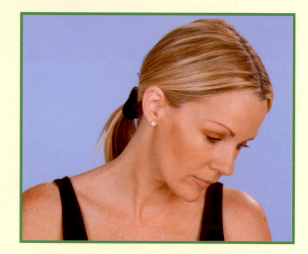

THE REAR NECK STRENGTHENER

This exercise helps to strengthen and stretch the back of the neck
to improve the head's proper posture, by toning the
sternocleidomastoid and *trapezius* muscles.

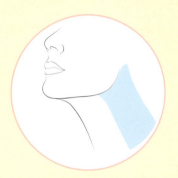

Put your head down as far as it can go and fully relax the muscles
in the back of your neck so that your head hangs forward.
Drop your shoulders and take a deep breath. Move your head
slowly from right to left 5 times while feeling the stretch from the
tops of your shoulders and relax. Repeat as necessary.

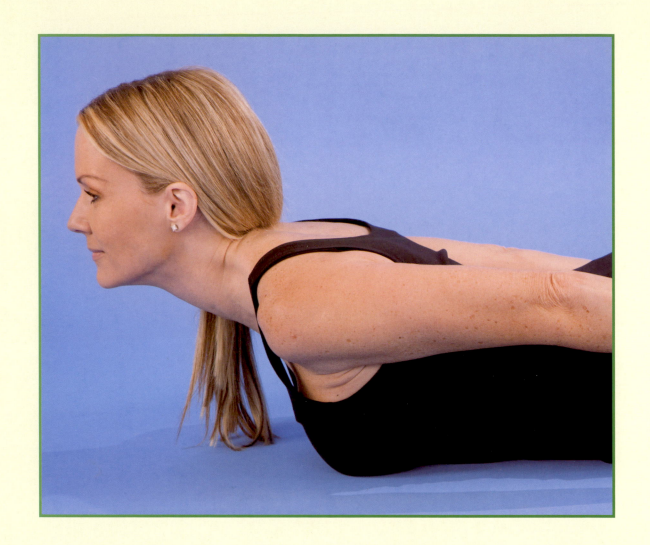

THE NECK STRAIGHTENER

"Text neck" is a very real and nearly epidemic condition caused by the horrible posture of our heads, necks, and arms when texting. This exercise will correct the forward tilt of the head and relieve the back pain caused by texting and extensive computer work. It will tone the *sternocleidomastoid*, *trapezius*, *occipitalis*, and *rhomboid* in the back of the neck. In the front of the neck, the *platysma* will get a nice workout.

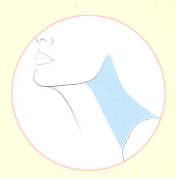

Lie on your stomach on the floor. Lift your head off the floor, look forward, and raise your arms upward behind you at your sides. Hold for 10 seconds and then relax. Repeat 3 times.

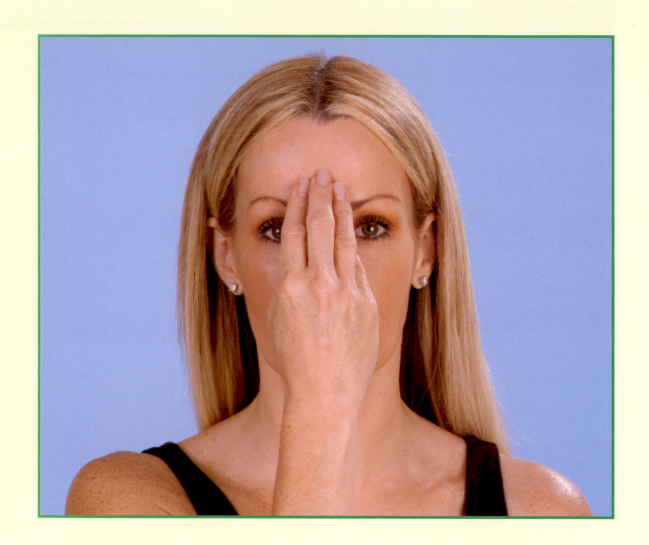

THE BETWEEN-BROW RELAXER

This exercise helps to alleviate the vertical lines between the brows and helps to prevent this area from drooping and creating a horizontal fold over the nose by toning the *nasalis*, *procerus*, and *frontalis* muscles.

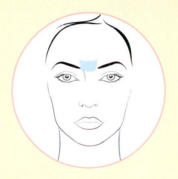

Press firmly with 3 fingers between your eyebrows just above your nose, concentrating on pressing down the tip of your nose, and hold for 5 seconds and then relax. Repeat 3 times.

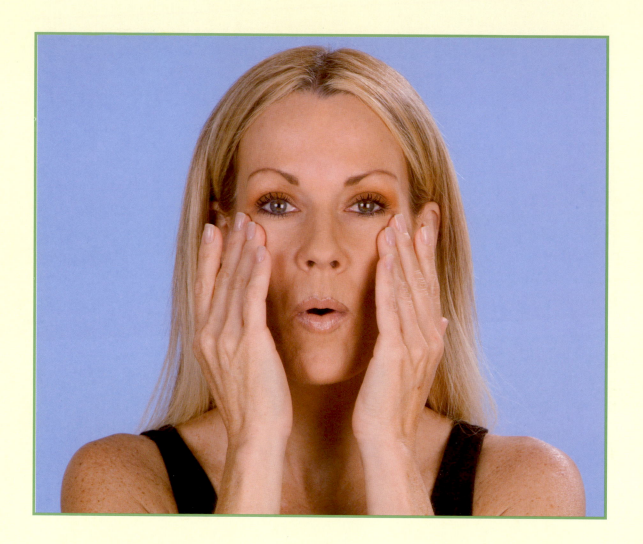

THE CROW'S FEET ELIMINATOR

This exercise diminishes the appearance of crow's feet near the eyes by building and plumping the muscles around the eyes so that the skin lies flat and smooth, even when you smile. It tones the *orbicularis oculi* muscles.

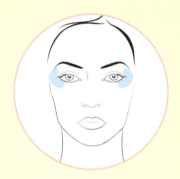

Open your mouth, making an "O" as wide as you can, and place your middle and ring fingers just below the outer corners of your eyes. Squint up into the inner corners of your eyes, trying to close your eyes using only the lower lids—keep upper lids still and open—pumping 10 times and then relax. Repeat 3 times.

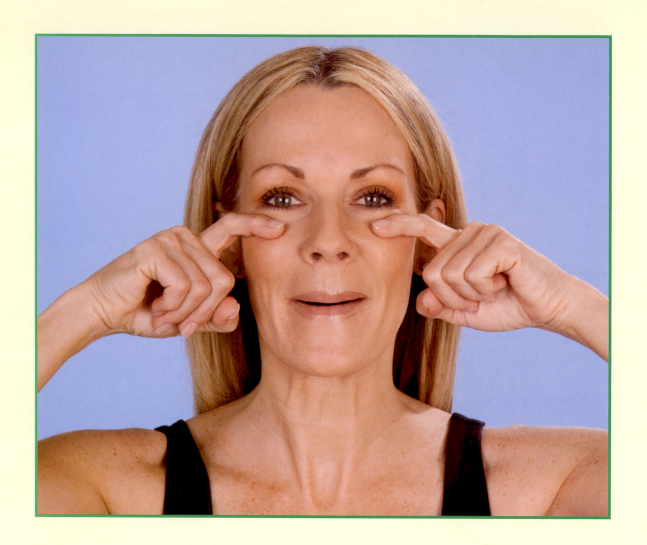

THE CHEEK PUSH-UP

This exercise prevents the cheeks from drooping and helps to eliminate excess facial fat by toning the *zygomaticus minor* and *major*, the *buccinator*, and the *masseter* muscles.

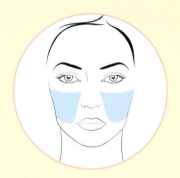

Open your mouth and roll your lips inward and under your teeth, then place your index fingers just above the apples of your cheeks. Pump your cheeks up toward your fingers 10 times, using your fingers for resistance, and keep your eyes quiet and still, then relax. Repeat 3 times.

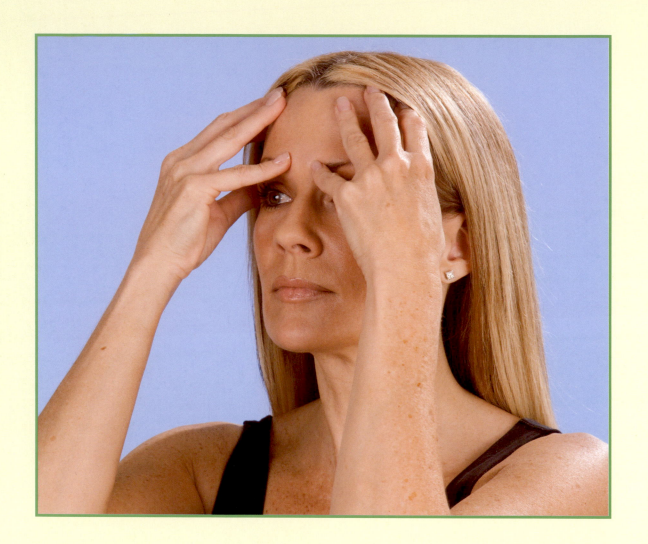

THE FOREHEAD RELAXER

The problem I find with the forehead is its over-use. It is far more effective to train the forehead muscles to relax in order to eliminate horizontal lines and wrinkles than to simply strengthen the muscles. This exercise helps to relax the entire forehead muscle instantly and provides a simultaneous massage using pressure points to relieve stress and tension by relaxing the *frontalis* and *procerus* muscles.

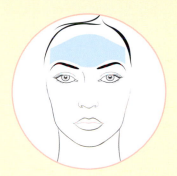

Place all 10 fingertips on and around the forehead in this order: pinkies just inside your inner eyebrows, your index, middle, and ring fingers up along your hairline, and your thumbs at your temples. Press your fingertips in while slightly rotating your hands for 5 seconds and then release.

CHAPTER 5

THE MASSAGE TECHNIQUES

MASSAGE has been practiced for centuries and is considered among the oldest forms of healing. With regular facial massage you can have firmer, smoother skin by increasing the skin's temperature, which causes the skin to release toxins and impurities that cleansers alone cannot reach. Beneath the skin's surface, massage enhances the action of the lymphatic system by moving bacteria and waste away from the skin cells so these toxins can be eliminated. Facial massage also strengthens and tones the facial muscles, and prevents wrinkling and sagging. Massage of the face and neck increases circulation by maximizing cellular turnover and brings nutrients to the skin's surface to give you a more radiant appearance. It is also very effective in helping to relieve stress. When you feel stressed, the muscles in your face contract. This often results in headaches, jaw pain, and even neck pain, and can cause deep wrinkling. Massage relaxes the muscles, releases tension, and helps to revive the spirit.

The primary concern regarding facial massage is the condition of the skin and the subcutaneous musculature—that is to say, the health of the outer skin and the underlying muscles. The idea is to work specifically and precisely within the facial meridian or acupuncture points to achieve a balance in the entire facial skin and muscles. The following massages use a variety of surface strokes as well as deeper pressure massage to work the musculature underneath the surface

tissue. Use these techniques to stimulate the nervous system, which increases blood circulation, reduces and prevents wrinkles, repairs and balances the condition of the skin, minimizes the aging process, and leaves your face looking and feeling fantastic.

Massage relaxes the muscles, releases tension, and helps to revive the spirit.

The Facial Fitness massage techniques were designed to complement the Facial Fitness exercises. You may perform these techniques after you exercise your face; however, it is recommended that you create a calm, serene environment in which to do the massages. Perhaps light a scented candle and play some soft music in the room where you're doing your massages. Before you begin the massage techniques, remember to thoroughly cleanse your face and neck and apply your facial moisturizing cream to both. Besides helping the fingers glide over the skin and ensuring smooth, even strokes, applying moisturizer minimizes the risk of stretching your skin.

To begin, warm a few drops of facial massage oil between the palms of your hands and start by holding your hands just below your nose and taking a deep breath to enjoy the aromatherapy of the oil.

Lavender is especially soothing and relaxing, as is rose and apricot oil when added to jojoba, sesame, or hazelnut oil. Apply to the face and neck as you do the massage techniques, always massaging upward to combat gravity.

Store your massage oil in a dark glass bottle in a cool, dark place, such as a cabinet. This will help keep its potency longer. Perform your facial massage while sitting or standing to help drain the lymphatic system and eliminate toxins. Like the exercises, you should do these techniques once a day for the first three weeks, and then you can downgrade to once every other day.

THE MASSAGE TECHNIQUES

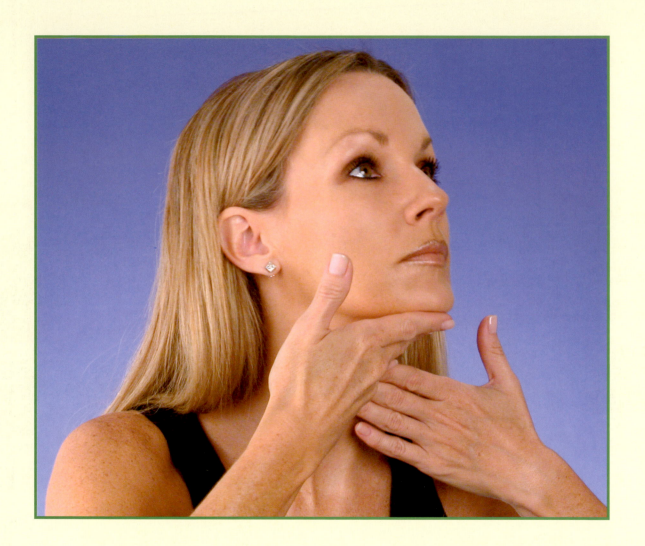

THE NECK SWEEP

This massage will increase circulation to the neck
and eliminate any puffiness.

While applying massage oil with your fingertips,
sweep in an upward and outward direction, beginning
at your collarbone and going up your neck with
your hands turned slightly outward. Cover your entire neck
while turning your head from side to side 5 times.

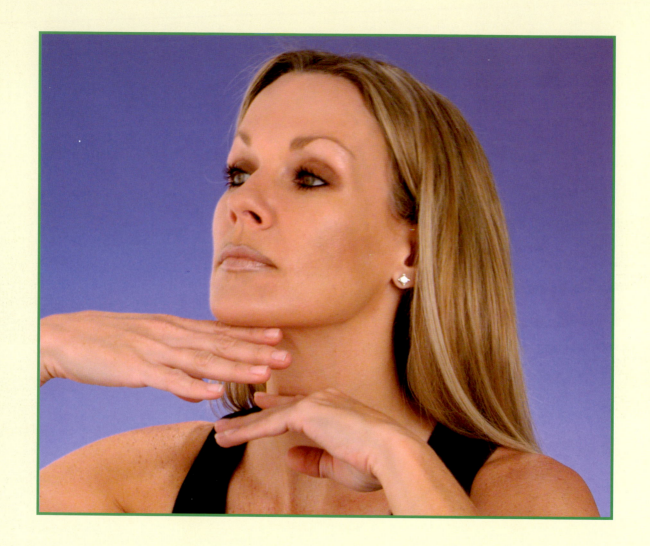

THE ADVANCED NECK MASSAGE

Like the Neck Sweep, this massage is designed to increase circulation and help rid the area of any fluid buildup.

With your hands open and your palms facing down, using the backs of your fingers, roll your hands forward under your chin, each hand following the other for 10 seconds. Repeat as needed.

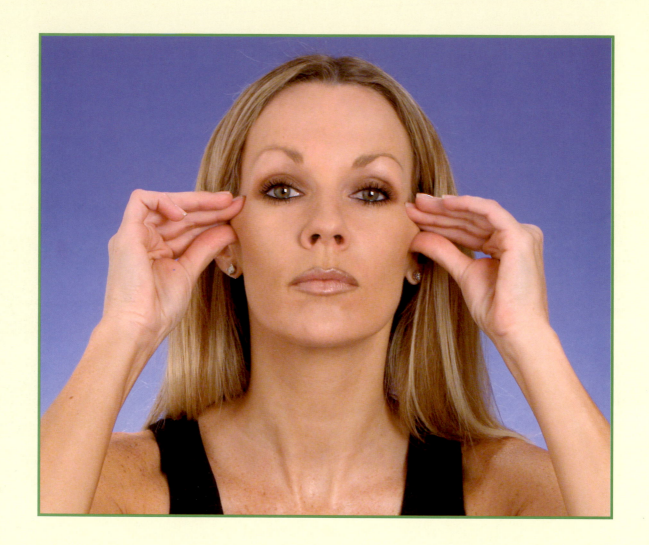

THE SKIN GRASP

This technique will help to rejuvenate the elasticity
of the facial skin.

Gently grasp your skin just above your jawline
with your thumbs, index fingers, and middle fingers.
Slowly, pushing up with your thumbs, grasp your skin,
creeping up toward your eye. Begin again at your
jawline, rolling up toward your ear. Around your forehead,
walk your fingers up around your hairline. Begin again
at the inside corners of your eyebrows, rolling outward
to each temple. Repeat as needed.

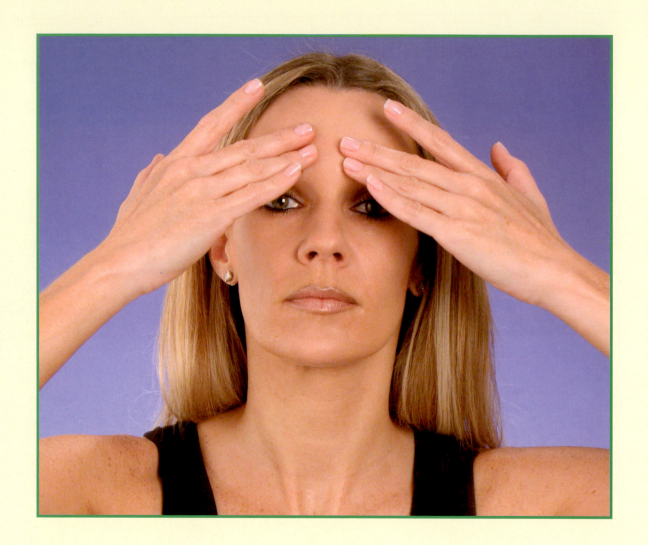

THE BETWEEN-BROW MASSAGE

This area of the face is the most prone to developing deep vertical lines. This technique helps to relax this area instantly.

With the tips of your fingers, gently massage the area between your eyebrows 25 times in a small circular motion. Repeat again in the other direction. Apply more massage oil, if necessary.

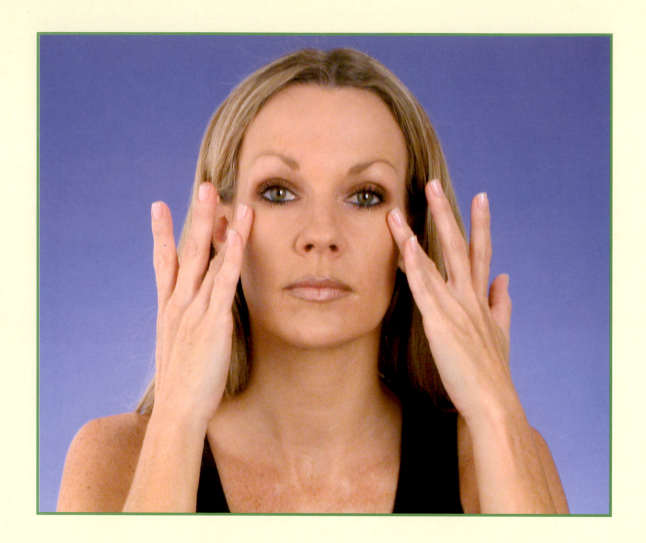

THE EYE AND BROW MASSAGE

This stimulating technique increases circulation and helps
to flush out built-up fluid around the eyes.

Apply eye cream with your ring fingers
(because they provide the lightest touch) to your eye area
in a gentle, tapping motion. Then, in a circular motion,
gently massage the area around your eye from the
inside to the outside, around and around, 10 times.
Finish by gently tapping under your eye to promote
circulation and reduce puffiness.

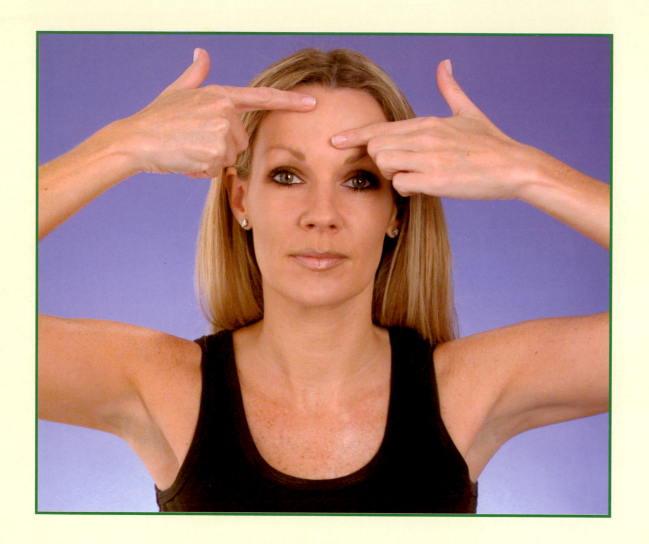

THE FOREHEAD MASSAGE

Much like the massage for the eyes, this will help to eliminate
any fluid buildup and relax the *frontalis* muscle.

With your fingertips, gently massage your skin,
making a semicircle on your forehead above your eyebrows.
Expand the motion outward toward the temple areas and back.
Finish by massaging the temple areas in a circular motion,
then stop and apply slight pressure to your temples for
a moment, and release. Repeat as needed.

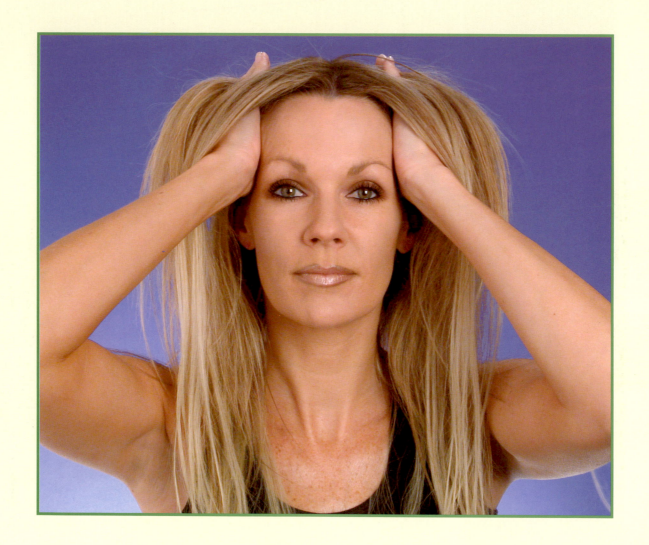

THE SCALP LIFT

This relaxing method of massage increases circulation to the scalp,
which will promote hair growth as well as relieve tension.

Place both hands under your hair on your scalp.
Gently lift your hair from the roots and hold
for 3 seconds. Repeat this technique all over your
scalp, making sure to cover your entire head.

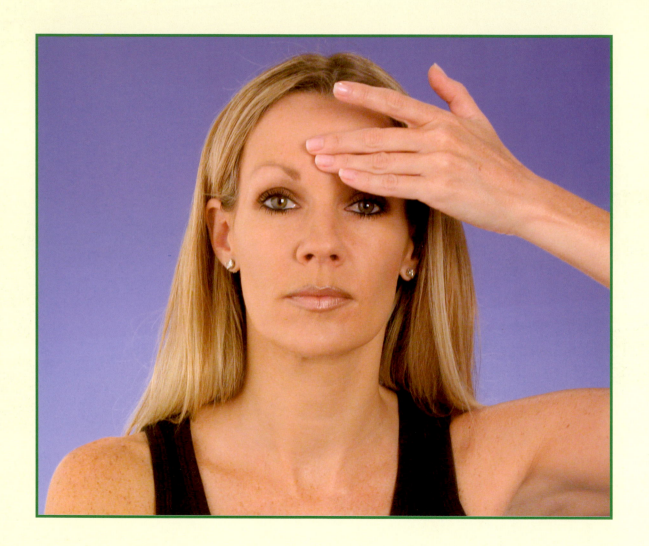

THE FROWN RELIEVER

This technique is designed to relax the muscles that
cause vertical frown lines to form.

Place your index and middle fingers just inside
your eyebrows. While applying slight pressure to the area,
gently sweep upward toward the center of your forehead
and hold for a moment while applying slight pressure
for 3 seconds. Repeat as needed.

This massage is recommended for the treatment of Bell's palsy.

THE MASSAGE TECHNIQUES

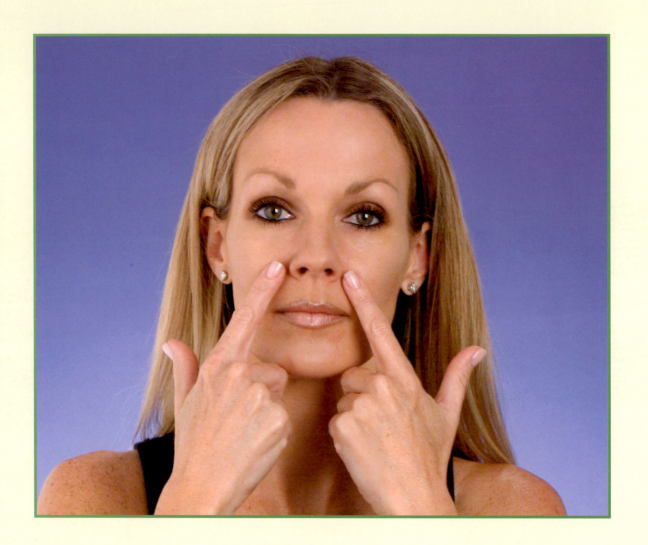

THE CHEEKBONE RELAXER

This massage increases facial circulation and
also helps clear the sinuses.

Starting at the corners of your nose, apply slight
pressure to your nose with your index finger. Sweep
out toward your ears and hold for 3 seconds.
Repeat as needed.

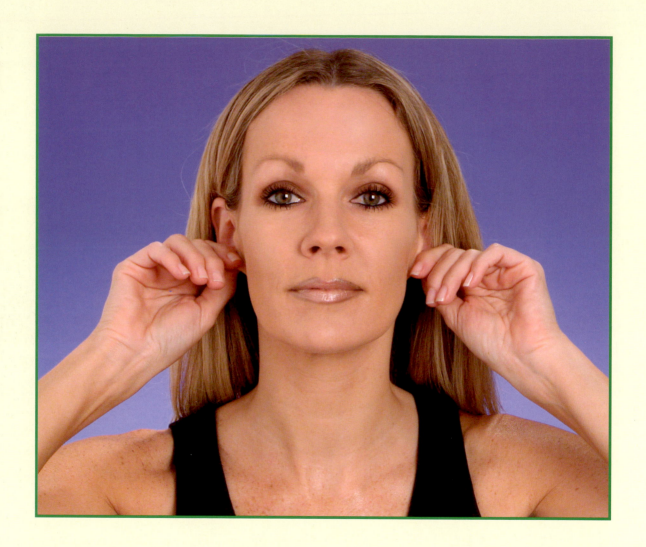

EAR TENSION RELEASE

This technique is great for relieving tension all over.

Starting at your earlobes, squeeze to apply slight
pressure and hold for 3 seconds. Sliding upward toward
the back of your ear, again apply slight pressure
and hold for 3 seconds. Finish at the top of your ear.
Repeat the cycle 3 times.

You may also pull backward gently on your ear
for more relief when you are finished.

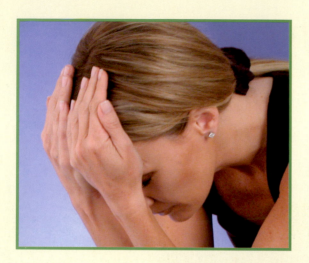

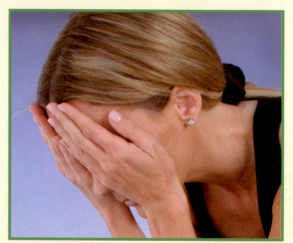

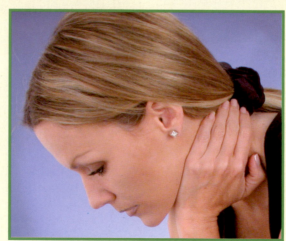

THE FACE PRESS

This massage increases circulation, eliminates puffiness,
and relaxes the muscles of the face and neck.

Sit down and rest your elbows on your lap.
Turn your palms up and rest your forehead on the
palms of your hands. Fully support the weight of
your head in your hands and relax your neck completely.
Breathe deeply and relax. Hold for 5 seconds.

Moving down to the eye area, place your
closed eyes in the palms of your hands and
relax completely. Hold for 5 seconds.

Now, move over to your cheeks and hold for 5 seconds.

Next, move down to your chin and jawline
and again hold for 5 seconds.

Finally, turn your hands outward and finish
with the front and sides of your neck, making sure
not to stretch the skin. When you are finished
sit up, breathe normally, and relax.

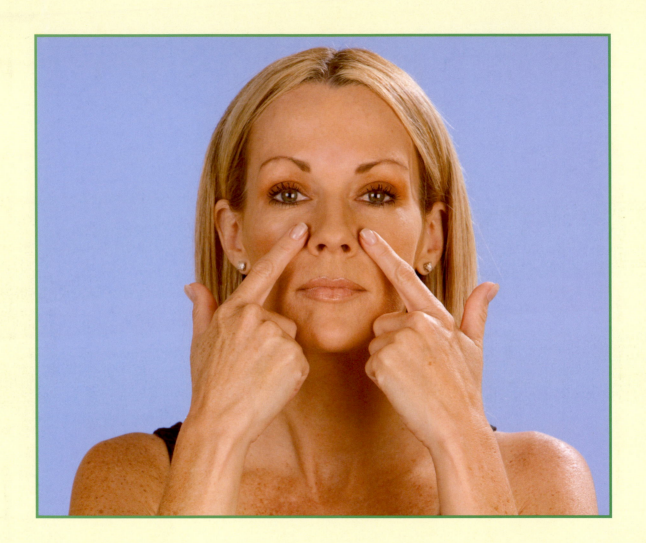

FACIAL FITNESS

THE NOSE MASSAGE

This technique will help eliminate any swelling around the nose and help with lymphatic drainage, which is the ability to effectively flush fluids and toxins from the body and, more specifically, the skin.

Using the tips of your fingers, massage from the bridge of your nose down and outward toward your cheeks 5 times.

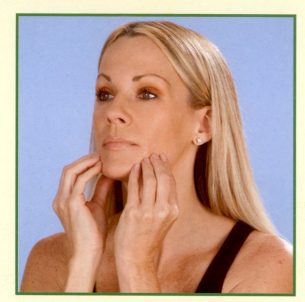

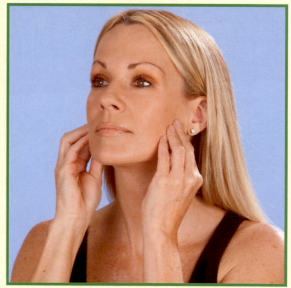

THE JAWLINE LIFTER

These techniques will tone and lift the jawline by activating collagen production
and increasing circulation, skin temperature, and blood flow,
which will immediately bring oxygen to the cells.

With your four fingers above your jawline and your thumbs
just under your chin, apply firm pressure and sweep your
fingers upward toward your ears. Repeat 5 times, always
beginning at the center of your chin and making sure
not to pull or tug on your skin.

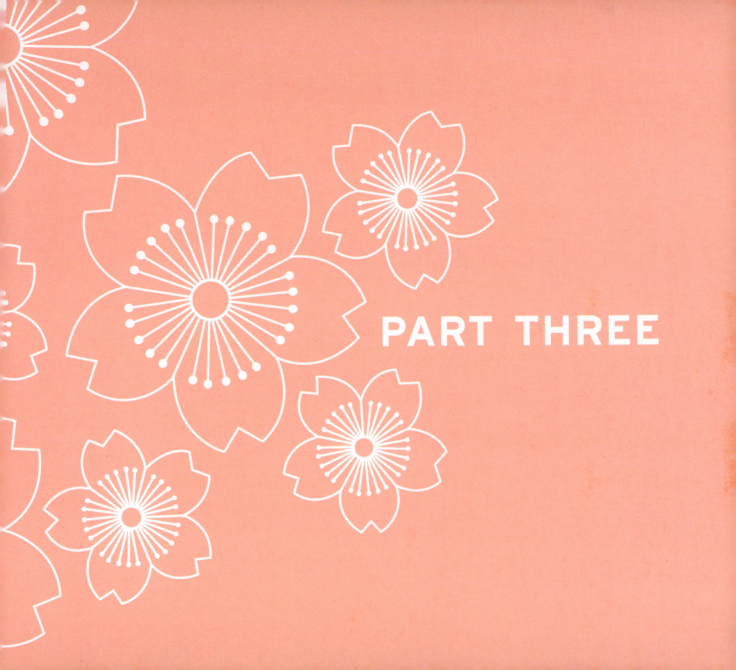

PART THREE

CHAPTER 6

HEALTHY LIFESTYLE, HEALTHY SKIN

IT'S NO SECRET that lifestyle choices greatly affect the way you look and feel. Your lifestyle has a critical impact on how your face and body show signs of aging. By making smart choices, you can significantly reduce the rate at which your skin begins to show these outward signs. By doing the Facial Fitness exercises and massage techniques, eating right, protecting your skin from the elements, and choosing beneficial skin-care products, you can stay looking fabulous well into your forties, fifties, sixties, and beyond.

As you may know, the skin is the largest organ in the body. It must have proper care and nutrition to carry out its vital functions. Primarily, the skin protects the internal systems of the body and acts as a barrier against the outer elements. It also helps keep you hydrated and regulates your body temperature through the sweat glands. It allows you to feel sensations like pain and warns you of potential harm. It's also a good indicator of internal health. For example, if your skin begins to turn yellowish, it may be an indication of serious illness, such as jaundice or liver cancer. So make sure you take care of your skin, because you only have one!

CLEANSERS, MOISTURIZERS, AND COSMETICS

Of course, you need to be as concerned about what goes onto your skin as you are about what goes into your body. Every substance that comes in contact with your skin that can be absorbed—and most can—reaches your internal organs in about twenty-six seconds. It is not just for the sake of your skin that you wash off potentially hazardous materials and liquids as soon as possible—it is because they are being absorbed deep within your body almost instantly.

Many large cosmetics companies use synthetic or petrochemical ingredients in their skin-care products.

Now think about what is in your cosmetics and skin-care products. Don't really know? Well, you had better start reading those labels more carefully. Many large cosmetics companies use synthetic or petrochemical ingredients in their skin-care products. Mineral oil, a by-product of the distillation of gasoline from crude oil, is one such ingredient, and is commonly used in lotions and baby oil.

Mineral oil and other petroleum-derived ingredients form a seal on the skin that traps moisture in but clogs the pores and prevents the skin from breathing and eliminating toxins. Mineral oil can also be harmful if ingested or inhaled, making it an especially hazardous choice for use on babies. Because of these dangers, the medical community has condemned the use of mineral oil taken orally or as an ingredient in medications. However, it is still available in many cosmetics and personal-care products, so let the buyer beware.

I only recommend and use skin-care products that consist of natural, plant-based ingredients and other essential nutrients.

Cosmetics and personal-care products containing animal products or by-products should also be avoided. Remains from slaughterhouses and other places where dead animals are collected after being killed are combined in one big vat and boiled down in what are called rendering plants. The fat and other substances are removed and then sold to large cosmetics companies. These then become key ingredients in the manufacturing of many products, such as lipsticks. I don't know about you, but I'm not putting that on my skin. I only recommend and use skin-care products that consist of natural, plant-based ingredients and other essential nutrients. They may cost a bit more, but for me—and for you—they are well worth it.

Some cosmetic and skin-care products contain carcinogenic or otherwise toxic ingredients that can damage your skin or be detrimental to your overall health. To learn more, I suggest reading a fascinating book by Christine H. Farlow, D.C., called *Dying To Look Good*. According to the book, some of the ingredients you should be aware of and avoid are:

- **Fragrances:** Each has up to six hundred different ingredients that may not be listed on the label.

- **Preservatives:** These may contain formaldehyde, which is a carcinogen, neurotoxin, irritant, and sensitizer.

- **Talc:** This is a known carcinogen and is not recommended for use on children.

- **Artificial colors:** Many of these cause cancer. D&C and FD&C colors are derived from coal tar, a known cancer-causing agent.

- **Silica:** While it is not harmful by itself, it may be contaminated with crystalline silica, which causes cancer.

❧ **Propylene glycol and sodium lauryl sulfate:** Common ingredients in shampoos, these are both skin irritants. If ingested, propylene glycol can cause kidney and liver damage, and sodium laurel sulfate degenerates cell membranes and can alter the genetic information in cells, as well as damage the immune system.

Dying to Look Good is a great reference that will help you identify hundreds of dangerous ingredients in well-known brands and guide you toward selecting safer products. Be smart and keep yourself informed by researching and finding the best products available to make you look your best, and steer clear of those with questionable ingredients. Here's a good rule to follow: if you can't pronounce it, you may want to avoid it.

Here's a good rule to follow: if you can't pronounce it, you may want to avoid it.

Now that you know some of the ingredients your cosmetic and skin-care products should not contain, here are a few of the beneficial ingredients that they should contain:

❧ **Retinoids:** Probably the number one secret to perfect skin is retinoids. According to Dr. Katie Rodan, the co-creator of Proactiv® Solution and Rodan + Fields Multi-Med Therapy®, "Retinoids work by getting rid of dead cells and turning over the cells more rapidly." Prescription-strength retinoic acids are used to fight acne, correct sun-damaged skin, and increase cell turnover. Retinol, which is the pure form of vitamin A, is weaker than retinoic acid, making it perfect for sensitive skin. Regardless of the formula you use, be prepared to go through a "worse before better period." Make certain to avoid sun exposure, especially when using these products, and wear a broad-spectrum sunscreen even on cloudy days.

- **Antioxidants:** Incorporating products that contain antioxidants, which are needed to combat the signs of premature aging, dehydration, and loss of tonicity, into your daily skin-care regimen is vital to the health of your skin. Look for products that contain vitamins A, C (L-Ascorbic Acid), D, E, B5, B6, B12, minerals, peptides, and hyaluronic acid.

- **Stem Cell Treatments:** Stem cells are specialized cells that act as the primary source of how every cell in the body develops. They can be "programmed" into skin cells, bone cells, and even tissue cells to repair damaged cells and replace them with ones that function properly. Now with the latest discovery that fat is rich in stem cells, "There is no controversy associated with these stem cells because they are sourced from your own body and nothing is harmed during the extraction process," says Beverly Hills plastic surgeon, Renato Calabria, MD. Stem cells can be used in fat transfer through injection, however, the procedure is not yet readily available in the United States because the device used in the procedure is not yet FDA-approved. There are, however, a number of products available that activate the stem cells you already have with ingredients that strengthen and prompt the production of new ones. When used daily, stem cells are protected, wrinkles are reduced, and skin appears to be more radiant.

Fruit Enzymes: The skin naturally exfoliates about every 28 days, but it can only shed so much on its own. Exfoliation is key in maintaining healthy skin, but some exfoliators can be very harsh on the face. Enzymatic exfoliators that contain enzymes derived from fruits such as pumpkin, kiwi, orange, and papaya are

Enzymatic exfoliators that contain enzymes derived from fruits such as pumpkin, kiwi, orange, and papaya are ideal for all skin types, including sensitive skin.

ideal for all skin types, including sensitive skin. They are gentle to the skin because they rest on the face with no scrubbing and are not irritating like some products containing beads or spheres, and they are very effective for cleaning out clogged pores. Each time you exfoliate you help remove the top layer of skin and diminish the appearance of discoloration and acne scars, restore a smoother texture, and reveal fresher, brighter, younger-looking skin.

Peptides: Hyperpigmentation is a common skin condition that occurs when more than normal amounts of melanin are produced, leading to dark pigmentation in the skin. The sun is the main cause of hyperpigmentation, but hormonal changes or a reaction to an injury (inflammation) like acne, eczema, or even a cut or burn, can also cause discoloration. Products containing hydroquinone have been used to diminish the appearance of hyperpigmentation, however, the potential toxicity associated with hydroquinone makes products containing peptides a smarter choice. Peptides contain amino acid chains that may be able to lighten these brown spots more effectively when they are small enough to penetrate the skin and be absorbed deep within the layers of the skin. There are a few products available that do just that, so research to find the one that is best for your skin type. Along with this treatment, wearing sunscreen on a daily basis is a crucial step in preventing and reducing hyperpigmentation.

DMAE: Also known as dimenthylaminoethanol, it is a phenomenal ingredient that helps protect skin cells and acts as an antioxidant, preventing damage from free radicals. Free radicals are atoms with an uneven number of electrons in their outer shell. This means that one electron is unpaired, making it chemically reactive, so the atom will now try to steal an electron from a neighboring molecule to stabilize itself. By stealing molecules from others, they in turn create more free radicals in the process. They damage healthy cells, especially those of collagen. The damaged collagen becomes stiff and is no longer flexible, so the skin begins to look old or damaged.

And More: Another beneficial ingredient is copper peptide, which helps heal the skin. EGF, or epidermal growth factor, is another amazing substance. This protein promotes skin-cell growth, creating firmer skin with regular use. Coenzyme Q10, another vitamin, is an antioxidant that also fights free radical damage in the skin cells. Alpha-lipoic acid is a fatty acid that fights free radicals and helps protect the skin. One of the most popular ingredients in skin-care today is vitamin C. However, make sure you look for products that say "stabilized vitamin C" on the label, or better yet, those containing vitamin L-ascorbic acid. Another fabulous ingredient that has been proven to fight inflammation, free radical damage, and irritation, as well as promote healing, is vitamin E, or tocotrienol.

All of these substances have been shown to be very beneficial to your skin. Each of these ingredients works in its own miraculous way to improve the skin's health, tone, and texture.

Products made from natural plant extracts or plant-based ingredients, without harsh soaps or chemicals, are better for your overall health and provide a greater benefit for the skin. They are readily available in the marketplace and are suitable for most skin types. But beware, just because it says "botanical" does not necessarily mean it is safe for all people to use. Some of the most toxic and allergenic substances in the world are derived from plants, so it is important to know what you are allergic to before you choose a new skin-care line. Read the label of every product carefully if you have any known allergies and test a small amount on a less conspicuous area than the face to make sure you are not allergic to it.

That said, many botanical ingredients have been proven safe and effective in helping to improve the skin's quality. Some botanical ingredients, such as green tea, aloe vera, ginkgo biloba, and echinacea have been shown to reduce inflammation in the skin. Green tea

Products made from natural plant extracts or plant-based ingredients, without harsh soaps or chemicals, are better for your overall health and provide a greater benefit for the skin.

contains powerful antioxidants. When taken orally, these antioxidants act as a natural combatant that contributes to healthy cells by absorbing harmful free radicals. When applied topically, such as in a cream, it does the same for the skin. Aloe vera, a plant that has been used for centuries to heal wounds, has been shown to improve overall healing and relieve skin irritations.

Skin-care products containing both vitamins and botanicals have been proven to enhance overall health and the appearance of the skin. Over time, they can even undo some of the environmental damage we suffer from toxins in the air and water by promoting healing and offering protection from environmental toxins.

As mentioned previously, it is also important to include a broad-spectrum sunscreen in your daily skin-care routine by either choosing a day cream with an SPF of fifteen or higher, or using sunscreen alone before you apply your other skincare products. The greatest skin-care products in the world won't make a difference if you continue to accelerate the aging process by failing to protect your skin from exposure to the sun. I cannot stress this point enough: don't leave home without sunscreen.

The greatest skin-care products in the world won't make a difference if you continue to accelerate the aging process by failing to protect your skin from exposure to the sun.

Your basic skin-care routine should consist of cleansing, toning, and moisturizing.

Remember to read labels so you can avoid products that contain harsh soaps or fragrances, and choose products that are formulated for your particular skin type, be it normal, oily, dry, or a combination of these. Use a gentle skin cleanser and try to cleanse your face twice a day. If you can only cleanse once a day, do it at night, before you go to bed.

Sleeping with makeup on your face is one sure way to get acne and dull skin. Consult with a dermatologist if you have a condition that may increase your skin's sensitivity, such as eczema, psoriasis, or acne. A gentle exfoliator used occasionally will help the skin look more radiant by removing dead skin cells. But it can also remove some of the protective cells from the skin's surface, so don't overdo it.

Not only does proper nutrition oxygenate the cells, but it provides the antioxidants needed to fight off attacks from free radicals that bombard you.

GOOD NUTRITION

As mentioned earlier, the skin looks its best when properly hydrated from within. Moisturizing is great, but most creams just draw water from within the skin's layers and hold it on top for a while. Drinking plenty of water, preferably distilled, will keep your skin looking great and your body functioning properly, because water provides a good infusion of oxygen to all areas of the body. Why is distilled water better? It is thought that distilled water is neutrally charged, or has no charge. Therefore, as it passes through your system it picks up those harmful free radicals and flushes them out more effectively than non-distilled water.

A few vitamin lines available today are specially formulated with high levels of antioxidants. These vitamins come in both pill and liquid form and have been proven to help protect and repair the skin from within. Look for formulations containing green tea, grapeseed, and beta carotene, and add these to your daily routine.

I cannot stress enough how important good nutrition is to the skin. By consuming the vital nutrients and vitamins needed for the body to thrive and repair itself, you are helping the skin cells regenerate faster. Not only does proper nutrition oxygenate the cells, but it provides the antioxidants needed to fight off attacks from free radicals that bombard you on a continual basis. A well-balanced diet, designed to bolster your overall health as well as the skin's appearance, includes oily fishes such as tuna, mackerel, and salmon, which are filled with beneficial omega-3 fatty acids and are excellent sources of protein. Skinless chicken, turkey, eggs, yogurt, and cheese are also excellent sources of protein. And let's not forget veggies. Green, leafy vegetables such as escarole, spinach, and arugula are all excellent sources of vitamins and nutrients. Avocado, asparagus, cauliflower, broccoli, and eggplant are bursting with vitamins, minerals, and antioxidants as well. Garlic has many health benefits, as do tomatoes and peppers.

Green, leafy vegetables such as escarole, spinach, and arugula are all excellent sources of vitamins and nutrients.

Some fruits to add to your diet are strawberries, cherries, kiwis, and blackberries. Choosing organic produce is always best. If organic produce is not readily available in your area, make sure you wash your fruits and vegetables thoroughly before eating or cooking, since many of them are treated with pesticides. Some fruits, such as strawberries, hold on to what they are treated with more than others, so be sure to wash them more than once. You should also consume strawberries shortly after you remove the green leafy stem, because once the skin is cut, the strawberry begins to lose its vitamin potency.

Some healthy snack alternatives are naturally dried fruits, nuts, olives, and raw vegetables. Of course, before you start adding any of these foods to your diet, make sure you are not allergic to them or intolerant of them. Another tip for good eating habits is to try to prepare foods with olive oil, as opposed to other types of oils or margarine, because it contains more nutrients. Always smell the oil before you use it; oil may become rancid, and rancid oil has a toxic effect on the body.

Try to cut down on the amount of sugar you eat. Besides promoting tooth decay and adding empty calories to your diet, sugar can also make acne worse. Chocolate, while not completely hazardous because of the benefits from the flavonoids it contains, should be kept to a minimum as well. Limit the amount of salt you use to flavor the foods you eat and avoid seasoned salts that contain MSG, because it may cause headaches.

Use butter or spreadable margarine (the kind that comes in a tub) in moderation, but avoid margarine and shortening that comes in stick form. These products undergo hydrogenation to turn them from a liquid to a solid, and to extend their shelf life. Hydrogenated oils—which are also found in fried foods, fast foods, pastries, cookies, and other snacks—contain high levels of trans fatty acids, which raise LDL ("bad") cholesterol levels and lower HDL ("good")

cholesterol levels, and increase the risk of developing heart disease and stroke.

Try to chew food on both sides of your mouth to prevent alignment problems with your jaw and teeth, and to maintain normal function.

It may seem like an odd thing to be aware of, but for those who want to avoid any potential problems with TMJ disorder, or for anyone currently suffering from it, you should try to be aware of which side of your mouth you are chewing your food on. Try to chew food on both sides of your mouth to prevent alignment problems with your jaw and teeth, and to maintain normal function. If you usually eat on the right side, try eating on the left side once in a while.

As you are probably aware, cigarette smoking is by far one of the worst habits you can develop. Smokers will tell you that smoking can quickly become an addiction that's not easily overcome. Besides the proven correlation between smoking and various cancers, emphysema, and other serious illnesses and diseases, smoking is one of the biggest causes of premature aging. The carcinogenic chemicals contained in cigarettes reduce the skin's elasticity. Smoking also creates an abundance of unchallenged free radicals, which accelerate the aging process, not to mention all the squinting and puckering going on whenever one drags on a cigarette. Just look at the

mouth of someone who smokes. The vertical lines surrounding their mouth are a telltale sign of years spent smoking.

The carcinogenic chemicals contained in cigarettes reduce the skin's elasticity.

PHYSICAL AND EMOTIONAL HEALTH

Aside from the products you put directly on your body or into your body, a number of other factors affect the way your skin looks. The position in which you sleep can greatly affect the way you look in the morning. Sleeping facedown with your face buried in a pillow will certainly guarantee a puffy, line-filled complexion. And sleeping on one side or the other will crease the face and cause lines that over time will become permanent.

Try to sleep on your back with your head slightly elevated on a pillow to reduce swelling or creasing on your face. If you must sleep on your side, position the pillow behind your ear and away from your face so that you are not creasing your face and causing permanent sleep lines.

Getting enough rest is one of the most important ways to help your body regenerate and heal, so make sure to get at least eight hours of sleep each night. Taking an occasional afternoon nap is also great. Getting just a few minutes of extra sleep in the afternoon will rejuvenate and recharge your batteries before you head off for a busy evening.

As practitioners of mind-body health have known for centuries, being happy is vital to good health.

"Never underestimate the power of laughter." Whoever said that first couldn't have been more correct. With all that you endure in a day, and all the challenges you face from moment to moment, it's a wonder how you manage to keep your sense of humor. But smile you must. First of all, smiling is good for your facial muscles. And don't worry if it causes lines around your eyes, just do your eye exercises and you'll look great. As practitioners of mind-body health have known for centuries, being happy is vital to good health. So try to surround yourself with happy, positive people and good friends as much as you can.

Laughing out loud with my friends, playing with my children, drinking great red wine, riding my horses, and being in love are all things that make me happy. Your idea of happiness may be entirely different, but remember that your personal happiness is the goal, so try to make time to do what you enjoy as often as you can.

Taking a walk daily can do wonders for the body as well as the soul. Take a few deep breaths and remember to swing your arms rhythmically to reeducate and balance the brain. It is great exercise and the endorphin release makes you feel fantastic.

Allow yourself to live life to the fullest and enjoy every minute by living in the present. Don't worry about mistakes you've made in the past or what may lie ahead in the future. Living in the present will make such a difference in how you look and feel, and it will make you much more attractive to those around you.

QUICK FIXES FOR THE FACE AND HAIR

So you just woke up and your face is puffy and tired-looking. It happens to everyone. Maybe you partied a little too much or you just couldn't fall asleep. Whatever the reason, there are a few things you can do to remedy this. First, start by taking a nice warm shower and thoroughly cleansing and exfoliating your face. Finish your cleansing routine by running cool water over your face and gently pat dry. Apply your toner and let it air-dry.

Apply your makeup sparingly, as it tends to settle into fine lines, making you look older.

When washing and especially drying your face, avoid rubbing the skin too hard. Try not to stretch the skin with your hands by rubbing your eyes when you're tired. As a matter of fact, try to avoid touching your face during the day as much as possible, because as you know, your hands are not always clean and the dirt and bacteria can cause breakouts.

After washing your face and applying your toner, apply your eye cream with your ring finger in a gentle tapping motion all around the eye area. Let each product dry for a few moments before applying the next one. Now, apply your moisturizer (one that contains one or more of the recommended ingredients) to your face and neck and do each of your Facial Fitness exercises. Follow that by doing all of the Facial Fitness massage techniques, except the scalp lift (we'll save that for later). This will help eliminate any fluid buildup that causes puffiness, especially around the eyes, and increase circulation to eliminate any toxin buildup. If your moisturizer does not contain sunscreen, apply some now. Apply your makeup sparingly, as it tends to settle into fine lines, making you look older.

If you wake up with a new addition to your complexion in the form of a mini–Mount St. Helens, here are a few tips that can quickly remedy the problem. When your skin breaks out, you should never squeeze the blemish before it is ready. This can cause swelling and terrible scarring. After thoroughly cleansing your face, you should apply heat, such as a warm compress, to bring the pimple to a head, and then apply a topical medication or clay mask to dry it out. You can also try applying ice to the pimple to reduce the redness and swelling. Ice causes blood vessels to shrink temporarily. Another good remedy to try is to crush an aspirin and add a drop of water to it to form a paste. Apply this aspirin paste directly to the pimple. Aspirin contains salicylic acid, which is the same ingredient found in acne-control products. Do not use this aspirin paste if you are allergic to aspirin.

Regular visits to the dermatologist can help keep acne under control and minimize the occurrence of breakouts. Your dermatologist can prescribe medications and treatments designed to prevent breakouts from occurring in the first place. I am a great fan of facials and find them to be beneficial for many reasons. First of all, they are a relaxing indulgence that I think everyone should experience. Secondly, they remove dirt, makeup, and built-up oils trapped deep within the skin and leave the face really clean. Finally, the rejuvenating facial massage is wonderful for the circulation and helps to release toxins built up within the skin's layers. Try to either get a professional facial at least once a month, or give yourself a facial at home. The extra care you lavish on your skin will show in both the skin's tone and its radiance. Just make sure you use quality products that contain pure ingredients. Many salons and spas have excellent products available for purchase so that you can achieve similar results at home.

Try to either get a professional facial at least once a month, or give yourself a facial at home.

To help get back that healthy look from within, start by drinking two or three glasses of water and a cup of green tea, if you have it. If you don't, it's time to go get some and add it to your daily routine. The antioxidants contained in green tea help rid the body of toxins, absorb free radicals, and decrease inflammation in the skin. Take a vitamin high in antioxidants and make sure to eat a breakfast rich in protein and nutrients, such

as egg whites, oatmeal, melon, and some fresh tomatoes. These tips will have you looking and feeling better in no time.

So what about that hair? Has it lost its luster and shine? Well, here are a few tips to help increase circulation to the scalp and bring back some of the shine that can be stripped away by overuse of hair-care products. While in the shower, shampoo your hair twice. Use a shampoo that is right for your particular type of hair, like a deep moisturizing formula if your hair is dry and brittle. It is a good idea to use a clarifying shampoo once a week to remove built-up residue on the hair left by styling products. Follow by applying a moisturizing pack containing protein and let it sit on your hair for a few minutes while you begin your skin-care regimen. Keep a wide-toothed comb in the shower and comb the conditioner through your hair before you rinse it out. Rinse your hair with cool water, with your head tilted back, to keep as much of the conditioner as possible off your freshly cleansed face. Wrap your wet hair gently with a soft towel. Apply a leave-in conditioner with detangler to your hair and comb it through to the ends. Style hair as usual, but before you apply any type of finishing product to the hair, such as hairspray, perform the scalp lift massage technique to increase circulation and relieve stress.

If you don't already own a bonnet dryer, consider investing in one. Once a week, apply a protein pack to your hair, or if you don't have one on hand, put olive oil into a spray bottle and spray your hair until it's saturated, cover with a plastic shower cap, and sit under the dryer for fifteen minutes. Thoroughly wash out the oil, and your hair will look and feel incredibly soft and shiny. Most beauty supply stores carry bonnet dryers and protein pack conditioners.

COSMETIC OPTIONS AND FACIAL FITNESS

The question has arisen on numerous occasions whether or not you can start exercising your face once you have had a cosmetic procedure, such as collagen or restylane injections. The answer is a resounding yes. According to the American Society of Aesthetic Plastic Surgery, cosmetic procedures consisting of filler injectables such as restylane have been steadily increasing from year to year. Because these injectable fillers do not cause partial paralysis in the facial muscles, as does Botox, the muscles can still be toned and strengthened effectively as an adjunct to these procedures.

Botox, or botulinum toxin type A, is a purified derivative of botulism. The purified toxin is diluted and directly injected into the facial muscles, restricting the ability to contract that particular muscle. Used primarily on the frontalis muscle and around the outermost part of the eye muscles, this temporary effect makes it somewhat difficult to effectively exercise these muscles. If you are doing facial exercises and want to continue to do so for the remaining muscles of the face and neck, by all means you may do so without worry of undoing the effects of the Botox. Incidentally, immediately after the Botox injection has been administered, it is recommended that the patient do facial exercises for at least two hours to help the Botox work more effectively.

This is not exactly what the Facial Fitness program was designed for, but if you do choose to go the Botox route, well then, there is one more way to use the facial exercises you have learned.

As mentioned earlier, plastic surgeons generally encourage the use of facial exercises both before and after facial cosmetic surgery as a way of enhancing and prolonging the effect of the procedure. So, if the surgical route is one you have already embarked on, or are considering embarking on, then you can make the Facial Fitness program part of your pre– and post–operative routine, if your physician advises you to do so.

CHAPTER 7

BEAUTY SECRETS FROM AROUND THE WORLD

F OR CENTURIES, WOMEN throughout the world have been trying to attain "beauty." Of course, beauty means different things to different people, and each culture has its own standard. However, there are certainly some universal ideas of beauty, and one of them is smooth, blemish-free, young-looking skin. Within different cultures, there are always some women who seem to know how to maintain and enhance their natural beauty by taking care of their skin better than others. What do they know that others may not? What secrets have been passed down from generation to generation that we might benefit from? One thing these cultures have in common is that, for centuries, women have have been using natural remedies to treat and prevent the effects of aging. The good news is that many of these beauty treatments are available to us as well, with a quick trip to the health food store. Aside from the convenience and ecological benefit of using natural ingredients, you will also save tons of money using these methods—no $300 face creams for you! Through years of travel, research, and interviews, I have compiled a diverse list of beauty secrets and tips from women around the world, and here are just a few that I would like to share.

FRANCE

French woman have long been revered as some of the most beautiful women on earth. Their emphasis on skin-care and diet is second to none, and, of course, we all know that Paris is the beauty capital of the world. Some of the finest skin-care products available on the market today are from France. The French's emphasis on natural, plant-based skin-care is at the forefront of the industry. However, there are some homemade recipes using simple, inexpensive ingredients that French women have been using for years to keep their skin looking healthy and young. Here are some of my favorites:

- To easily remove eye makeup, gently apply **sweet almond oil** using a cotton pad to the delicate eye area. Not only does it remove the makeup entirely, it also moisturizes and protects the skin. You can also use sweet almond oil during facial massage before cleansing.

✿ ✿ ✿

Aside from the convenience and ecological benefit of using natural ingredients, you will also save tons of money using these methods—no $300 face creams for you!

✿ ✿ ✿

✿ Mix natural **powdered clay** with water to make a thick paste, then apply to the face and body. Let dry and rinse off thoroughly. It will help draw out impurities in the skin and reduce pore size.

✿ To minimize puffy eyes, apply **chamomile tea bags** that have been steeped and cooled to the eyelids for five to ten minutes. Chamomile is a natural anti-inflammatory, which helps to dissipate fluid build-up.

You can find sweet almond oil, powdered clay, and chamomile tea at your local health food store.

RUSSIA

Russian women know a thing or two about combating rough, dry skin due to the harsh Russian winters. They have developed a few natural remedies to soften their skin and keep it young-looking and supple, as well as blemish free. Here are the remedies I have found to be the most effective:

✿ To accelerate cellular turnover and keep your skin looking young, apply skin-care products containing **caviar**. Fast cellular turnover occurs naturally in women in their twenties and thirties, but once you get older, you may need some help. It is thought that caviar interacts with the skin at a cellular level, producing faster cellular turnover, and helps keep the skin looking supple, hydrated, and youthful for years to come.

Use **arnica flower**, which grows in the mountains of Siberia, to combat bruises. It increases circulation and stimulates white blood cells to fight the bacteria around the bruise. Look for products such as creams and gels that have arnica as the main ingredient at your local health food store.

ISRAEL

Within this remarkable ancient land lies one of the most coveted beauty secrets in

Fast cellular turnover occurs naturally in women in their twenties and thirties, but once you get older, you may need some help.

the world: the **Dead Sea**. The Dead Sea is the lowest spot on earth and is also the richest in concentrated natural minerals, making this area a world-renowned natural health destination. The curative properties of the Dead Sea have been recognized since the days of King Herod over 2,000 years ago. For centuries, people have traveled to this destination for what was thought to be its mystical healing powers. Cleopatra traveled from Egypt to build the world's first spa there. "Today we know that the Dead Sea contains 35 percent of minerals per liter of water," says Ziva Gilaad, chief cosmetics director of AHAVA, a major packager of Dead Sea skin products. The concentration of over 21 different minerals contained within the water is believed to help such skin problems as eczema, psoriasis, joint pain, arthritis, and fluid retention.

Often referred to as the biggest natural spa on earth, the Dead Sea waters naturally contain clay and minerals that are absorbed into the skin and draw out deep impurities, and which cleanse, moisturize, and promote new cell growth. As the mud dries on the skin, it thoroughly pulls out all toxins from the pores while infusing the skin with a high concentration of minerals and

The Dead Sea is the lowest spot on earth and is also the richest in concentrated natural minerals, making this area a world-renowned natural health destination.

nutrients essential for healthy skin. It also acts as an exfoliant because of the fine grains present in the mud that peel back layers of dirt and dead cells to reveal younger, more radiant skin.

If you can't make it to the actual Dead Sea, there are several product lines available in the United States containing mud from there, but Dead Sea Laboratories LTD (D.S.L.) is the only Israeli cosmetics firm with exclusive rights to extract the mud and sell raw materials from the Dead Sea. These products are marketed under the brand name "AHAVA" and have won three international awards to date. You can find them in many stores, or online at www.ahavaus.com.

The curative properties of the Dead Sea have been recognized since the days of King Herod over 2,000 years ago.

JAPAN

Japanese woman have the most incredible skin: flawless, poreless, and toned. What is their secret? The answer is facial massage and a cleaning process called **The Oil Cleansing Method**. Daily, they use oils such as castor oil to draw out dirt and other impurities from their pores, and extra virgin olive oil (EVOO), which is a brilliant moisturizer, to help heal and nourish the skin. Here's how to use this exceptional secret to your advantage:

For normal skin, combine one part EVOO to one part castor oil in a small bottle and shake. For oily skin, combine three parts castor oil to one part EVOO, and for dry skin, combine one part castor oil to three parts EVOO.

To begin, pour a quarter-sized amount of the combined oils into your palm, rub your hands together, and slowly massage your skin using the techniques in Chapter 5. Do not wet your face first; apply the oil dry. Work the oil into your skin for about a minute and enjoy the peaceful massage. Don't scrub, just massage.

Next, wet a washcloth with hot water (not scalding) and place it over your face for a few moments until it begins to cool. This will steam out your pores, removing the impurities and the dead skin cells.

Finally, thoroughly rinse the washcloth with hot water, wring, then gently wipe off any excess oil. Your skin will feel softer, look brighter, and won't feel tight or greasy. Olive oil has the same pH as human skin so it is the perfect cleansing balancer. You may not even need a moisturizer. I use this cleansing method at night and in the morning, and my skin looks rested and bright.

Olive oil has the same pH as human skin so it is the perfect cleansing balancer.

SWEDEN

These fair-haired beauties are very familiar with the fact that the sun can wreak havoc on their skin, and they also know how important relaxation is in keeping their skin young and wrinkle-free. They have quite a few tricks up their sleeves to take care of their skin, but here are the best Swedish methods:

❧ Aside from using sunscreen daily, they take **rose hips** to combat wrinkles from collagen breakdown due to vitamin C deficiency. It helps keep the complexion smooth and healthy looking by fighting the damage caused by free radicals produced from excessive UV exposure. You can find rose hips at your local health food store.

🌸 Keep skin glowing and minimize pores by splashing your face with **cold water** after cleansing.

🌸 **Swedish massage** has been performed for centuries and is based on the theory that massaging in the same direction as the returning flow of blood to the heart helps to relax the muscles. The light pressure and rhythmic stroking helps to create a level of relaxation that is so profound it's hard to stay awake.

GREECE

The Greek goddesses know a few things about beauty and natural remedies to treat and heal the skin from head to toe. According the owner of By The Strand Salon and Spa in Weston, Florida, Rita Molfetas, Greek women have several all-natural remedies that anyone can use:

🌸 Use a combination of plain **Greek yogurt and honey** to create a mask for the skin. Applied to the face and neck, it helps to exfoliate, tone, and tighten the skin, and also leaves it velvety soft. Leave the mask on for five minutes and then rinse.

🌸 Use pure **watermelon** as a toner, applied with a cotton pad. Let dry and then rinse.

- To make a fabulous body scrub, combine **olive oil with sugar** and rub all over while in the shower.

- To treat dry feet and cracking heals, dip feet in **warm olive oil** and then scrub with **sea salt**.

UNITED STATES

The United States is home to women from many different cultures, many of whom brought beauty secrets from their home-lands with them. There are also many clever homegrown American beauty tips and remedies.

- Take one tablespoon of **apple cider vinegar** in the morning to boost your metabolism, help digestion, prevent constipation, and make your skin look fantastic. If you have difficulty taking it straight, mix it with a glass of distilled water.

- Want an instant facelift? Try putting liquid **Pepto-Bismol** on a cotton pad and applying a thick layer to the face and neck as a mask. Leave on for about five minutes until it dries. Then use a washcloth moistened with hot water to gently remove the mask. Next, rinse your face with a splash of cold water. Amazing! The salicylic acid gives you a fabulous face peel, exfoliates the top layer of dead skin, and tones and tightens the face instantly!

- Is your skin looking tired and dehydrated? Try an **avocado mask**. Avocado is rich in fatty acids, vitamins, and protein, and is great for hydrating the skin. Mash one up and mix it with two tablespoons of Greek yogurt and a touch of honey to create a mask. Leave it on for five to ten minutes, then rinse. Your skin will perk up immediately.

Avocado is rich in fatty acids, vitamins, and protein, and is great for hydrating the skin.

🌸 To plump up your kisser, try dabbing a few drops of **cinnamon oil** on your lips. It will stimulate blood flow and instantly give you fuller, more youthful looking lips for hours.

🌸 Use **witch hazel extract** as a toner and quick skin pick-me-up. Mix one part witch hazel with two parts rose water in a small spray bottle and spritz your face to refresh tired, dehydrated skin. You can find both ingredients in a drug store or a health food store. I use this toner every time I fly, but make sure it's less than three ounces to carry it on board.

🌸 To add amazing shine to dull, lifeless hair, apply a small amount of **olive oil** to your hair, starting with a scalp massage and working it out towards the ends. Cover your hair with a plastic shower cap and sit in the sun for ten minutes. If you are in a colder climate or if it's winter, sit under a bonnet drier or blow dry (over the shower cap) on a low warm setting for a few minutes. Then, shampoo as usual.

A great leave-on overnight mask is a combination of two tablespoons of **plain yogurt** (I prefer Greek yogurt) and the juice of half a **lemon**. Mix and apply to your face and neck in an even layer, avoiding the eye area. Leave it on overnight if you can. In the morning, rinse your face thoroughly and it will feel silky smooth.

 For baby smooth skin, combine one cup of **sea salt** and half a cup of **olive oil**, mix well, and store in an airtight container. Use in the shower, after cleansing, as a great, inexpensive scrub. Avoid any open wounds or cuts and do not use internally or on your face. For added relaxation, add a few drops of lavender oil to the mixture.

Use a quality, broad-spectrum sunscreen or a skin-care moisturizer that contains sunscreen of at least SPF 15.

And last, but not least, probably the number one beauty tip that I hope is no secret to anyone, anywhere, is to use **sunscreen, every single day**. I cannot stress the importance of this enough, so it bears repeating. Use a quality, broad-spectrum sunscreen or a skin-care moisturizer that contains sunscreen of at least SPF 15. Remember to reapply it throughout the day if you are going to be out and about. It will help to prevent sun damage and the telltale signs of premature aging.

No matter where you are from, you can benefit from these time-tested beauty secrets. Please, make sure you are not allergic to any of these ingredients before you begin. Food sensitivities are very serious and can cause some very unpleasant side effects. Once you are sure you are allergy free, head to your local health food or grocery store and start saving money and improving your skin naturally!

CHAPTER 8

FINAL COMMENTS

THE TECHNIQUES AND TIPS I share with you in this book are designed to help you look and feel your best. By following a daily regimen of exercise, massage, good nutrition, and healthy lifestyle choices, you can reverse some of the visible signs of aging. With continued dedication to yourself, you will start to see the changes happen right before your eyes. People will begin to ask what you are doing differently and will want to know your secret. This proven method of toning and tightening the facial muscles will make you look years younger. And it only takes a few minutes a day.

With continued dedication to yourself, you will start to see the changes happen right before your eyes.

Good health and beauty start with a commitment to yourself, and a belief that you are worth it. To look and feel your best, you must make changes in your daily routine. For some, these are small changes, for others, this may mean changing everything. You should avoid habits and behaviors detrimental to your health and start making smart, well-informed choices. After all, it's never too late to make yourself a priority. Not only will the knowledge you gain be beneficial to your health, but to your children's health as well. You are your children's greatest teacher, so educate yourself about the potentially dangerous ingredients contained in many of the products that are on the market today and search for healthy alternatives. The Facial Fitness program was designed to be just that—a healthy alternative.

Incorporating all the essential components to healthy living into your daily regimen will guarantee that you look and feel your best, and it will show first and foremost on your face. You can achieve so many benefits from exercise and incorporating the Facial Fitness program into your daily routine, and this program will ensure that you keep your most visible asset looking great. It's never too late to start exercising your facial muscles. You are guaranteed to see results at any age.

Consistency is the key, so don't give up if you don't see results immediately.

As I mentioned earlier, because the muscles of the face are smaller than most, they respond to exercise rather quickly. Just remember to stick with it. Consistency is the key, so don't give up if you don't see results immediately. Remember: it took a lifetime to look the way you do now, so be patient and diligent, and soon you will begin to see an amazing transformation.

It has been my pleasure to share this information with you and I hope you will share it with others. Please refer back to this book and to the others I have recommended when you need inspiration, information, or simply to refresh your memory.

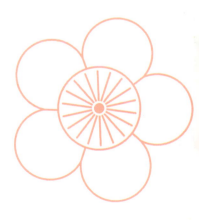

BIBLIOGRAPHY AND ADDITIONAL RESOURCES

The American Society for Aesthetic Plastic Surgery: http://www.surgery.org

Begoun, Paula. *The Beauty Bible.* Seattle: Beginning Press, 2002.

Bell's Palsy Research Foundation: http://www.bellspalsy.com

Colbert, Don, MD. *Toxic Relief.* Florida: Siloam Press, 2003.

Farlow, D.C., Christine. *Dying To Look Good: The Disturbing Truth About What's Really In Your Cosmetics, Toiletries and Personal Care Products . . . And What You Can Do About It.* California: KISS For Health Publishing, 2006.

Herbal Luxuries, "Mineral Oil and Why You Should Avoid It," Herbal Luxuries, http://www.herballuxuries.com/mineral-oil.html.

Lowe, Nicholas, MD. *Away With Wrinkles.* New York: Marlowe and Company, 2005.

Mochizuki, Shogo. *The Art of Japanese Massage.* Colorado: 1999.

Mohammed, Renea. "Animal Rendering Products In More Places Than You Think." *Animal Writes: The Vancouver Humane Society Newsletter.* Summer 2003.

Mitchell, Sandi, Ph.D. "Beauty, Pride and Pig Grease." *Health Freedom News.* Jan/Feb 1991.

Oxenreider, Tsh. "How to Clean Your Face Naturally," Simple Mom. http://simplemom.net/oil-cleansing-method/

"Retinol," *New Beauty Magazine.* Winter–Spring 2010.

The TMJ Association: http://www.tmj.org

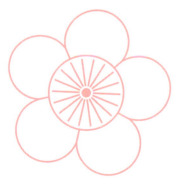

INDEX

Caviar, 167–168
Cells
    life span of, 21
    oxygen for, 137
    replenishment of, 27
    shedding, 22
    turnover, 108
Cheekbone Relaxer (massage), *128,* 129
Cheek Push-Up (exercise), *102,* 103
Chemicals, exposure to, 26
Chocolate, 155
Cholesterol, 155
Cinnamon oil, 174
Circulation, 21, 28, 31, 32, 113, 114, 129, 137
    massage and, 14, 107–108
Clay, powdered, 167
Coenzyme Q10, 149
Collagen, 22, 23, 27, 137
Colors, artificial, 144
Corrugator muscle, 42, 57
Cosmetics, 142–152
Cronin, Gaye, 33, 34
Crow's feet, 22, *100,* 101
Crow's Feet Eliminator (exercise), *100,* 101

D

Dehydration, 26, 146
Depressor septi muscle, 43, *45, 47,* 61, 83
Diet. *See* Nutrition and diet
Dilator muscle, 43, *47*

DMAE, 148–149
Double chin, 23, 73, 87, 93
Dying to Look Good (Farlow), 144, 145

E

Ears, elongation, 23
Ear Tension Release (massage), *130,* 131
Echinacea, 150
Eczema, 148, 152
Elastin, 22, 27
Emphysema, 156
Epidermal growth factor (EGF), 149
Estrogen, 23
Exercises, 28
    advanced, 80–105
    basic, 56–79
    for Bell's palsy, 34, 35, *60,* 61, *62,* 63, *64,* 65
    benefits of, 30–37
    breathing during, 52
    cheek, *102,* 103
    chin, *86,* 87
    eye, *76, 77, 78, 79, 88,* 89, *100,* 101
    facial, 14, 15, *58,* 59, *90,* 91
    forehead, *56,* 57, *74, 75, 98,* 99, *104,* 105
    jawline, *68,* 69, *70,* 71, *72,* 73
    lip, *64,* 65, *84,* 85
    mouth, *62,* 63
    neck, *66,* 67, *70,* 71, *72,* 73, *92,* 93, *94,* 95, *96,* 97
    nose, *60,* 61, *82,* 83
    physical, 158

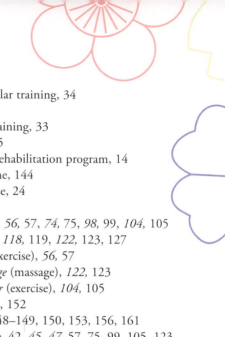

copper peptide in, 149
cosmetics, 142–152
Dead Sea minerals, 168–170
epidermal growth factor in, 149
facials, 160
fragrances in, 144
in France, 166–167
fruit enzymes in, 147–148
in Greece, 172–173
hazardous, 142, 143, 144, 145
hydroquinone in, 148
ingredients in, 11
international, 164–176
in Israel, 168–170
in Japan, 170–171
mineral oil in, 143
natural ingredients, 144, 150
Oil Cleansing Method, 170–171
peptides in, 148
petrochemicals in, 142, 143
preservatives in, 144
proactive, 28
propylene glycol in, 145
protocols
retinoids in, 145–146
routine, 151–152
in Russia, 167–168
silica in, 144
sodium lauryl sulfate in, 145
with sunscreen, 26

in Sweden, 171–172
talc in, 144
in United States, 173–176
Skin Grasp (massage), *116,* 117
Skin rejuvenation, 14, 15
Sleep, 156–157
need for, 24
Smoking, 24, 26, 156
Sodium lauryl sulfate, 145
Stem cell treatments, 146–147
Sternocleidomastoid muscle, 44, *47,* 67, 95, 97
Stress
alleviation, 14, 28, 108
effect on skin, 26
massage and, 108
Sugar, 154–155
Sun
exposure, 22, 24, 43, 146
photoaging and, 24
skin damage from, 22, 24, 25, 26, 146
UV rays, 22, 24, 26
Sunscreen, 24, 25, 43, 151
broad-spectrum, 26, 175
Surgery, cosmetic, 13, 14, 16, 162–163
pre-and-post operative exercise and, 16
Sweet almond oil, 166

T
Talc, 144
Tea

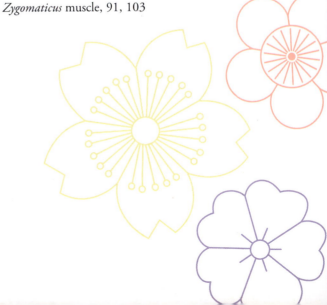